ONE *for the* COYOTES

*How I survived 40 years of my dream job
in TV news (and cancer too)*

Al Wallace
WDAF-TV Sports
1985 - 2018

AL WALLACE
with David Smale

D1707639

Foreword by BILL SELF

outskirts
press

I dedicate this book to my mother, father, and seven brothers and sisters. I also dedicate it to the most important women in my life now, my wife Marlena, and two daughters, Chase and Chaney.

Table of Contents

Introduction

IT'S ONE OF the best things about having a family, or being a part of a family. We're all able to laugh at each other, and ourselves. At least that's the way it is in my family.

My wife Marlena and I are blessed to have two daughters, Chase and Chaney. The four of us share a lot of love, but also at times, we teeter on the edge of getting on each other's nerves. It's what families do when they spend so much time together, and Lord knows we spend a lot of time together.

We all give each other a hard time about things we all find funny or distinctive. Over the years for me, it's been the inability to start reading a book and finishing it in timely fashion. By timely, I mean, years. At present, I've got three books in my nightstand that I've started within the past three years, and I've finished reading none of them.

Why not, you may ask? The reason is simple: time. I haven't had time. I'll start a book with good intentions, and then came the pull of my job in television sports broadcasting. Year after year after year.

The origins of writing this book began sometime within the past three or four years, I can't remember exactly when. I do remember being at Kauffman Stadium in Kansas City, waiting on Royals Manager Ned Yost to hold his daily press briefing for members of the media before a home game.

Standing and talking to a few other reporters and photographers, the subject of the infamous "Pine Tar" game came up. Among the group of scribes involved in the conversation was David Smale, who told us all that he and his wife were at that game in Yankee Stadium back in 1983. They watched in amazement as George Brett stormed out of the dugout and charged at home plate umpire Tim McClelland.

I remember that part of the day more than I remember who the Royals played, or even if they won or lost. I also recall that David asked me that day, in a private moment afterwards, "Have you ever considered writing a book?" It was one of those questions that I discounted almost immediately. I mean, I was too busy giving scores and editing sound bites. Where would I find time to write a book, and what exactly would it be about?

Well, over the next few years from time to time, I'd see David at different sporting events, and we'd share a hello or a brief conversation. At some point during that time period, we also became friends on Facebook. It wasn't until after I made the decision to leave television broadcast news and sports, that David reached out and messaged me on Facebook with a single question that I had never heard before in my life: "Are you ready to write that book now?"

This time, there was a solid connection and consideration. Within weeks, we agreed to meet for coffee and give the idea more than just a thought. 'One for the Coyotes' offers my perspective of 40 years in broadcast television, and my love for the history and perspective that it has helped provide to my life. That history included a number of positive accomplishments and setbacks. If I've learned nothing else, it's to learn from those ups and downs, through the history they have supplied to my life. They are true-life lessons I hope I've helped pass on to others, and to you. I sure hope you enjoy it.

So, with a lot of help from David Smale, I not only started a book, but I finished a book. As a byproduct, my family now has one less thing to kid me about or hold over my head. They are my heart and my soul. I dedicate this book to them.

Foreword

IF YOU'RE GOING to work at your craft, and part of your craft is building relationships with players, recruits, family or media, you should try to enjoy what you do. I learned early in my career that I didn't have to be buddies with the media, as far as dinner dates or doing things socially. But I have enjoyed getting to know them and things about them, and, in turn, opening myself up to the point where they feel like they know me.

Al Wallace is obviously well-thought of in local media, but to me he's been the face of Kansas City sports media since I've been here. There have been other regulars, but when I think of sports television in Kansas City, I think of Al Wallace.

I've always thought Al was professional, but I never thought it came with a win-at-all-costs attitude. He worked hard, and he was understanding and appreciative of my time. That made me want to help him if I ever could. When you have people who treat you well, you develop a connection with them. You don't have to go around telling everybody about it. It's kind of an unspoken thing. I know he's one of my guys and I'm one of his guys.

I always knew that Al enjoyed being over here. Maybe he just enjoyed his job so much that he enjoyed being anywhere. But I always felt like his disposition here was never about doing a job that he *had* to do. He enjoyed doing it. That's not easy when you're coming over here on a Tuesday afternoon before a Wednesday night game to talk with somebody in a hallway.

He always made me feel like it was the most important thing he could be doing. He told me about his affection for KU because his daughter went here and he met his wife here. But the extent of how much of a fan he is, I never would have known because he's such a pro.

I always enjoyed seeing Al and his main photographer, JW Edwards; if you saw JW, Al was there, and vice versa. When I saw JW in Omaha during the 2018 NCAA tournament, I said, "Hey, where's your guy?" He told me that Al's sister had died and that he wouldn't be there. I texted him and we corresponded by text for quite a while. I didn't feel obligated to reach out to him. That was just something you do for someone you like who is going through a hard time. That was just something you do when it's someone who means something to you.

I don't watch a ton of television. When I do watch something, other than ESPN, it seems like if I was watching the news, I always tried to tune in when I knew that Al was doing sports. So many young journalists believe the way you make a splash is to be controversial. I never felt like Al did that. Al would report the facts, and the facts would determine how he reported it.

Whether it was covering the Royals when they were on their two-year run in 2014 and 2015, covering the Chiefs when they were doing well, or even covering us when we've been on some good runs, I believe that Al got enjoyment from the local teams being successful. You could tell that from his reporting. It was always down the middle, but it was positive.

Al did his "dream job" for more than 40 years. I can just imagine all the things that he saw. I think you will enjoy reading about the behind-the-scenes things that nobody knows. We only see the obvious. He's seen what's not obvious. Al certainly knows how to tell a good story. This book is full of those great stories. Enjoy them like I have.

Bill Self
Head Coach
University of Kansas Men's Basketball

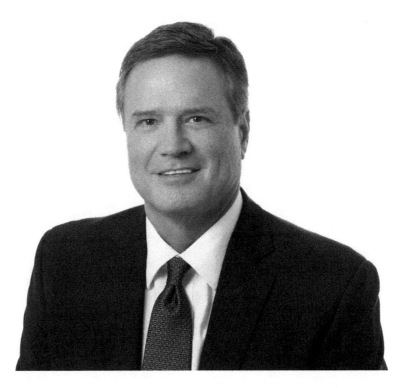

Bill Self

Acknowledgements

NO ONE GETS through the game of life without a lot of help, and for me, I mean *a lot of help*. This book, and the stories that make up my life's path, are only possible because I had assistance from so many people. I'd first like to thank my parents, Casper and Mildred Wallace.

I never knew a day in my life when they weren't working or concerned with making the lives of each one of their children better. My father had a lot of rules that led down a path that he thought was positive and right. He was the first in line to follow every single one of them.

My mother was the perfect example of love. She was caring, giving and had a great ear. I can't think of anyone ever saying anything negative about her. I thank them both for being shining examples of parenthood.

My brothers and sisters, Beverly, Lillie, Carlos, Jacelyn, Tony, Jada and Stephan. We were all Wallace kids. Our father wanted to make sure everyone who knew us knew being a Wallace was something different and special. We were not necessarily better, but certainly unique and good. I thank you all for your love and support, and for making each and every one of us feel like none of us were better, but certainly unique and good in our own separate way.

To Stephan, you will always be my *little* brother. Your counsel, your guidance, your friendship and your dependability mean so much to me. I thank you for all the years of love and support.

Thank you, Kathy Kuluva, for loving Stephan and being his soulmate. His happiness and security with you gives me comfort each and every day. You have no idea how much your togetherness brings peace to my heart.

On the television side of things, Bill and Stacy Jones, I thank you for being a great example of "till death do we part." Your friendship, your relationship and your marriage have been great examples of what a husband and wife, and father and mother, should be. Bill, working with you in Lubbock made being a teammate fun, enjoyable and important. I continue to cherish those years.

Mike and Cheryl McDonald, I survived in the industry as long as I did, mainly because of you. For some reason, you had faith in me. Mike McDonald once told a general manager, when speaking of me: "That guy will walk through a brick wall for you." I consider that the highest compliment a news director could ever say about me. Thank you.

Thank you, Thermal Stewart. I could always come to you for financial advice, though your job description didn't involve most of what you helped me with.

David Smale helped me write this book, and he helped me realize how much pleasure I could get out of writing and sharing my story of perseverance. David, thank you for your leadership and patience in helping me with this project. I thank your wife, Tammy, and your mother, Carol, for loaning you to me, and for their support and assistance.

Around the office at WDAF, my life and job were more comfortable, more efficient and much easier because of the efforts of newsroom personnel like Winona Murray, Tommie Luke and Kim Stripling. You all did so many little things over the years, too many to count, that helped me get through so many sportscasts, so many days, so many years in and around broadcast television. I can't thank you enough.

You can't last 40 days, much less 40 years working around television sports, without building trust and friendships with so many in the local sports community, especially those who work with high schools, colleges and professional teams. The list of those people I'd like to acknowledge and thank comprise a very long list. Among those that stand out are Dean Buchan, Chris Theisen, Jim Marchiony, Gary Heise, Mike Swanson, Brad Gee, Bob Moore, Pete Moris, Alfred White, Chad Moller and the late Bob Sprenger.

I'd like to thank every producer, director, manager, reporter, anchor, editor and/or photographer who had to put up with me being *me*. If you ever worked with me, you know exactly what I am talking about.

Finally, I'd like to thank my family: my wife and two daughters: Marlena, Chase and Chaney. The three of you are perfect for me, and I thank you and love you for making it that way.

CHAPTER 1

History

I AM AND always have been a family guy, probably because I grew up in a big family. It's all my mother ever wanted, and that's what she got: a big family and eight kids. I had three brothers and four sisters. I have a younger brother and younger sister, everyone else is older. My given name is Alva, though while I was on the air in television, I was referred to as Al. Most of my coworkers called me Alva around the office. I was named after my mother's oldest brother.

I grew up in a military family. My father grew up very poor, born in Asheville, N.C, which is also the hometown of former Kansas basketball coach Roy Williams. I'm a product of my parents and I'm a product of a military family. I grew up with structure: both from the Church of Christ and from my father, who was a sergeant in the U.S. Army. He also worked in a Civilian Conservation Corps, right after the Great Depression.

My father was born in 1915, the son of a brick mason, and barely graduated high school. He worked odd jobs before joining the Army at the age of 25. He spent one tour of duty in Korea and two tours of duty in Vietnam.

He did whatever he had to do to provide for his family. Sometimes he worked three jobs. He had a regular job in the Army, but if he had to work in the officers' club busing tables, or if he had to deliver pizzas at night, that's what he did.

During my lifetime, I've known a number of young people who grew up in broken homes. They didn't know who their father was or maybe when their father was going to be home. I didn't have to worry about any of that. I guarantee you my father was home 15 minutes after he left work.

It was always a laughing point around the family. When my father left for work in the morning, if he told you to have something done when he got home, there were no excuses. You knew he'd be home at 5:15. You could wait until 4:00 to do the task, knowing he was going to be home at 5:15.

The thing is, if the task wasn't done when he got home at 5:15, his wrath and his discipline was directed not only toward you, but toward the rest of the kids in the family. Everyone else would look at you and say, "You had this whole day, why didn't you do what you were supposed to do?"

That line of thinking forced me to grow up with a tremendous amount of discipline. It also melted into the rest of my life. I didn't always pay attention when I was a kid, but it was an obvious incentive.

It was also a tremendous help in my broadcasting career, because you have to have discipline. There are deadlines in broadcasting, sometimes several in one day. You have to be dedicated and you have to be accountable. If you don't do your job in broadcast news, others will suffer the consequences. You're not only accountable to your audience, you're accountable to your co-workers, and to the idea and responsibility of the free press.

How could you not do the job on time, and with integrity? You knew that sports went on the air at 10:20 p.m. There were no options. You knew there was a game. How could you not be there to cover it?

So, I'm a product of my parents, Casper and Mildred Wallace, and more than just physically.

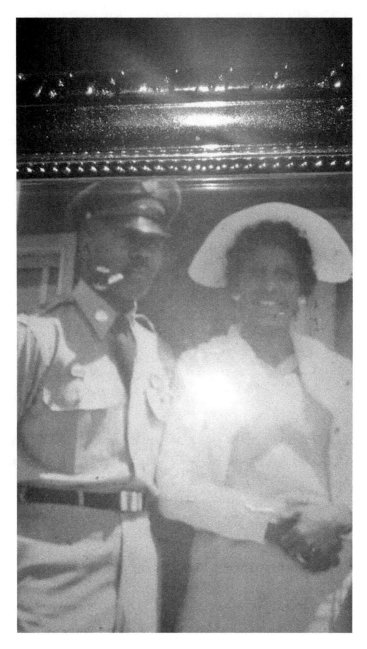

Alva was the sixth of eight children born to Casper and Mildred Wallace

A person can be a positive product of their parents or a negative product of their parents. I feel like I listened to all the positive things that they wanted me to be and do, and those traits outweighed the negatives. I totally believe that they would be proud of who I became. They're no longer with us, but when they were, they told all their children how proud they were of us. I still think of that. I know that before they both passed away, they were happy with what I had become.

Being a part of a large family with strict discipline and high expectations, I learned the value of sharing and teamwork. That would apply not only in working with a group of people in the newsroom, but also a smaller group of people in the television news sports department. Without question, it helped me in covering team sports. I knew how important teamwork could be, just from having seven siblings.

Second to my wife Marlena, my best friend is my little brother, Stephan. I still call him my little brother. He's six years younger than I, but he's still my little brother. He and I are so close because my two older brothers and I were not so close after our early teens. My oldest brother made some negative life-decisions, and he was an example of what I didn't want to be. That forced me to be a better big brother to Stephan.

We're all products of our environment, and part of my environment was growing up in the 1960s. I wondered at times if I'm unusual. Somewhere in the 1960s I knew I was living "history." I didn't say, "Oh, 50 years from now the 60s are still going to be this noteworthy decade," but I did realize events happening in the world around me were significant, very significant.

I remember in November 1963 when the secretary at my elementary school came into my first grade classroom. She was crying. Visibly shaken, she said, "The President has been shot." I had just turned 6 years old. When I got home that day, my Mom was on the phone trying to get in touch with her mother in Greenville, Texas, east of Dallas.

I remember a Sunday night in July 1969, running around in the backyard, when Neil Armstrong and Apollo 11 landed on the moon. I was 11 years old, and I looked up at the moon to see if we could see him. I thought out loud, "He's right there!"

Earlier in that decade, in 1964, we had moved to Germany and lived on an Army base in Darmstadt. For three years, I never got more than 17 miles away from my home. Living on an Army base in Germany in the mid 1960s was like living on an island. Imagine today never being more than 17 miles from home. I used to drive 17 miles to WDAF every day from my home in Overland Park, Kansas, sometimes twice a day.

While living in Germany, we were confined. I knew what Germany was, and I knew about the Berlin Wall, but we never got close to Berlin.

We knew the geographical and political climate we lived in could be dangerous. We had air-raid drills at night. We didn't have television. As a family all we had was a radio from our stereo. We could listen to music. Every once in a while, we'd get something from the Armed Forces Network or maybe a Christmas broadcast. Most communication you'd think we might have in the United States, we simply didn't have.

We did, however, have each other, not just as a family but as part of a community. I talk about my parents and some of the values that they thought were important for us to live by. Be loyal to your country because we're Americans here. If you wander off the Army base, you're not sure what's out there. My parents, and most military families, I believe, rarely saw any difference between Black and White skin color.

While in elementary school in Germany I went on a few field trips. We went to the zoo once. I remember German kids looking at me like I was an exhibit. The color of my skin was so different. These were German kids who didn't know any better, because they had never seen anything this different. They had never seen a Black person, much less a Black *kid*. I absolutely knew that it was different from living in the United States.

Of course, things back in the States weren't always great either. I started kindergarten at Fort Meade, Md., in 1962, and I went to school with White kids. In between the time at Fort Meade, and moving to Darmstadt, we moved back to Mineral Wells, Texas, near my birthplace at Fort Wolters, for a few months. That's when I went from an integrated school to a segregated school, and the difference was more than just visual.

We moved in with my great aunt. There were 12 of us living in a three-bedroom home. When we were in Fort Meade, we could go anywhere we wanted to go. In Texas in 1964, a simple thing like going across the street had to be thought through, because some White people might not want us there. When I was at Dunbar Elementary School in second grade, everyone was Black. Mrs. Holliman was my teacher. My best friend was Clarence Holliman, her son. Going to school there was different than school at Fort Meade, and I knew it.

It's hard to pinpoint how my affection for history has impacted my career. I do know it's offered perspective, including the knowledge that little things add up to big things. Ask former Chiefs linebacker Dee Ford if an insignificant foot makes a difference. He lined up a foot off-sides late in the fourth quarter of the 2019 AFC Championship Game. On that play, the Chiefs intercepted New England quarterback Tom Brady. Had Ford not been off-sides, the Chiefs would have gone to the Super Bowl.

What you do in life and what you do in a game, it's all significant. The little things add up and ultimately become important. That's part of what makes history significant.

When I watch sports, for work or just for fun, I see players, coaches and games. I like watching the journey they are on. People used to ask me why I didn't try to go to ESPN or work at a network. The fact is, I liked following the journey of a local coach, a person or a team throughout a season. I liked the journey that they go on from the first day of practice to the last day of a season, where they either did or did not accomplish their ultimate goal.

To me, that journey is their history. The best thing about it is, win or lose, they have another game the next day or maybe the next week. They get to write another chapter in their history. They can play another season.

I was out running errands the day after the Chiefs lost the AFC Championship Game in January 2019 to the Patriots, following my last year in broadcasting. I saw Royals Hall of Fame broadcaster Denny Matthews. As badly as I felt for the Chiefs and all of Kansas City for losing that AFC Championship Game, seeing Denny reminded me that Kansas City's got another chance.

It's all part of history; it's part of the cycle. We can't rewrite history, but we can absolutely try to make our history better the next day. That's part of the story I tried to tell with my live reports from the field, or my sportscasts on the anchor desk.

History isn't just about the events, it's about the people involved in the events. It's also about taking responsibility for the path we all take, and the decisions that we all make.

My first day on the job at WDAF was May 8, 1985. A few months later, I was at Arrowhead Stadium at the Truman Sports Complex in Kansas City. It was a normal day with John Mackovic as the Chiefs head coach. It was in the middle of the week, but I was among a number of reporters waiting to conduct player interviews. A guy came up to me and said, "Oh, you got the sports job opening at WDAF back in April or May."

I said, "Yeah." He said, "That's the job I wanted. You got my job." I replied, "No, *I got my job.*" He was blaming me for getting the job he wanted. I felt he should blame himself for not getting the job, which turned out to be a negative for him. I simply looked at it as a positive for me.

I feel it's all about responsibility and accountability. If I did a bad job of editing the highlights, or I did a bad live shot, I have no one else to blame. I'm the one who ultimately is accountable for the roof over the head of my family and the food on the table that feeds my family. I got that line of thinking from my parents.

Events don't carry the impact without the people involved with them. When I tried to tell a story on the air, I tried to "people-ize" the story.

I would tell our sports interns all the time, "I don't care if you watch SportsCenter every night. I don't care if you know the results of every game. When you tell a story or when you give information over the air, I hope that sports-geek who listens to sports-talk radio understands it and likes it. But we're also going for that grandma in Kansas City, Kansas, or that non-traditional sports fan. That person is more likely to understand people. It's likely they won't understand the stats and the metrics."

It's always important to connect with people. That's what I always tried to do. That's one of the reasons that I hope and believe strongly that everyone can connect with history, because everyone has a history. Some history is just more interesting or entertaining than others.

Our understanding and acceptance of each other's history is how we learn to respect each other and live with each other. That's the best thing about history. I believe sports is a tremendous "connector" to our lives.

It's very rare to hear a person traveling from one city to another saying something like, "How's that Ford plant doing in Kansas City" or "You've got 17 different coffee houses in Kansas City, right?" More often they might say, "With Mahomes, the Chiefs almost made it." or "That young QB is good." The teams, the players, the coaches, they travel the country, they play for a few months, and they represent the community.

The Ford plant and the coffee houses, they stay local. These players and coaches and teams connect us all. So when I tried to tell a story, I tried to understand the people or explain who the people were. When it comes right down to it, we're all the same, because we're all people.

We just have different histories.

If we recognize that history is about people and the events they help comprise, we most often interpret the significance of that event differently than the next person. We each have our own history to bring into the equation, and we each can interpret something different from an event.

My favorite example is a personal one, very personal. There was a football game at the University of Kansas on November 24, 1991. Most people remember that, in that game, Kansas running back Tony Sands rushed for two NCAA records: 58 carries and 396 yards. The fact that the opposing team was Missouri probably makes it a bigger deal for Kansas fans. There are probably plenty of people who recall a lot of details about that game. I'm certainly one of them, but for a different reason than most.

There was one elevator to the press box back then, a cranky old thing. Before kickoff, I got on the elevator with photographer Don Proctor, a Mizzou grad, and Lori Calcara, a KU student. Lori was one of the dance girls for the basketball team, and, at the time, a WDAF sports intern.

The three of us got on the elevator—a tight fit—and I saw Marlena Brohammer for the first time. She was the elevator operator.

I immediately fell in love. I trust that I did take my eyes off her, but I don't think I did. We got off the elevator and went to our seats in the press box. I turned to Lori, and said, "Did you notice the girl on the elevator?" Lori answered, "Yes, I noticed her, and I noticed that you noticed her."

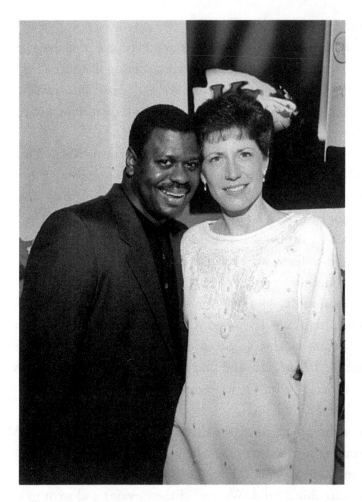

Al was captivated by Marlena the first time he saw her

During those days in gathering television news, with a lot less technology than we have today, we would have to get an engineer to park a microwave truck on a hill near Memorial Stadium in Lawrence. Memorial Stadium lies between two hills, so the engineer had to park on a hill behind the press box or a hill on the other side of the stadium.

To get highlights back to the TV station, the photographer had to shoot the game, then have someone get that video tape and take it to the microwave truck and beam it back to Kansas City and have it for the 5:00 news. That game was not televised, so that's the only way we could have highlights. For most games, that duty was assigned to the intern. On this day, I gladly took the assignment.

For most games, we would have to get those tapes to the engineer at the end of the first quarter or at halftime to cue up the plays and beam them back. That task took time. You missed part of the game, especially as slow as that elevator was. To keep up with the game, you'd better have a transistor radio or Walkman with earplugs to keep up.

On that day, I must have made 10 trips on that elevator running tapes, just to see Marlena and to say something. She lived in Overland Park and had a regular job working for the American Hospital Association. Being born in Lawrence and growing up on a farm near Baldwin City, Kansas, she liked KU athletics and she liked going to games.

I don't know if I said anything to her on the initial ride, but she knew she had caught my eye. If you ask her today, she will tell you that she knew I was looking at her. She absolutely knew something was up.

When I got home that night, I told my brother, "I met my wife today."

I didn't see her again for almost two months. It was late-January or early-February, when I saw her at a KU basketball game. She was working at a table where students came in and showed their IDs. I just happened to find her that day. So I went over and said hello and she said hi. She was still there after the game, so I approached her.

I didn't say, "I'm asking for a friend of mine," but I wasn't real pushy either. I simply said, "I saw you at a football game and I see you at this basketball game. So what if someone wanted to get in touch with you away from some KU sports venue, how would they do that?"

She didn't give me her phone number, but did say, "If someone wanted to do that, they could show up at StreetSide Records on 95th and Metcalf, by the Glenwood Theater in Overland Park. I work there

Sunday afternoons." She wasn't opening some door, like "Here's my phone number" or "Here's where I live." She just said, "Here's a public place. If you want to come in, buy a record and say hi, fine."

That next available Sunday, I went in to StreetSide Records and there she was. It was not like it was a hot, summer day, but I came in wearing sunglasses. How dumb. We laughed about that again very recently. I mean, what idiot does that?

Apparently, something worked, because we've been married for 23 years. We dated for about a year before she even allowed me to kiss her. We actually didn't really connect until 1994, after we had been dating for a couple of years. I had gone home to visit my mother in Texas, who was sick with esophageal cancer. I went to the hospital in Fort Worth and saw her. I couldn't believe it. She didn't look like the same person, and I knew the end for her was near.

I called Marlena. I remember being on a pay phone, crying, knowing my mother didn't have long to live. When I got back from that trip, Marlena was there for me. Our hearts melted together.

I'm sure Tony Sands remembers November 24, 1991, with fondness. It might be one of the greatest days of *his* personal history.

I know it sure was for me.

CHAPTER 2

A Product of the 60s

I BELIEVE THE 1960s were the most significant decade of U.S. history since the Civil War. The list of events that helped shape who we are now happened in that decade. The Cuban Missile Crisis in 1962, the March on Washington by Dr. Martin Luther King Jr.in August 1963, then the assassination of President John F. Kennedy just three months after that.

Later in the 60s came the escalation of the War in Vietnam, followed by the unrest it caused back here in the United States. Then, in 1968, the assassinations of Dr. King and Senator Robert Kennedy, followed a year later by the first man landing on the moon. These are all events that shook the very foundation of our country. Most people I know who were alive then probably can tell you where they were when each of those events happened. They certainly shaped who I was and who I have become.

I don't think you really know how any event, big or small, impacts your life until later, until it becomes part of your history. There are some who say history never ends, it simply evolves and continues. You can count me among that group.

I didn't see the 1960s as substantial in my life, until the early 70s.

That's when I began to realize those events didn't just affect my life, but they also affected the country and the world we all lived in.

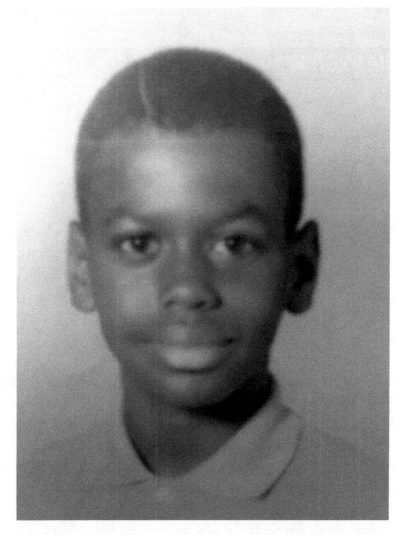

Al's outlook on life was shaped by growing up in the 1960s

I started my freshman year of college three months after I graduated high school in 1975, majoring in telecommunications at Texas Tech.

I minored in history. While in high school, I could already feel the influence of change the decade of the 60s had brought. So many things had happened and had a close, if not immediate, impact on my family.

Let's take these in chronological order, beginning with the Cuban Missile Crisis in October of 1962. We lived in Fort Meade, Md., less than an hour away from Washington, D.C., our nation's capital. My father was a sergeant in the Army. During the crisis, he, like many other soldiers, was deployed to the Florida Keys for emergency duty. The entire country, the entire world, was on edge. I remember the nervousness that enveloped my mother. The crisis never led to war, but my father didn't return home to Fort Meade until mid-December. Nine months after his return, my younger brother Stephan was born.

During the summer of 1963, I remember my mother and my oldest sister, Beverly, having a week-long discussion and dispute. Beverly was 14, and kept saying, "I want to go!" I was only 5-years old at the time, and I had no idea what the fuss was all about. I did know it involved a school-sponsored field trip, and my mother kept saying no.

My mother said there was no way she would allow Beverly to get mixed up in that "stuff." That "stuff" was the gathering of more than one million people. It was Dr. King's March on Washington. Beverly wasn't allowed to go. Even now, decades later, she still feels connected to it. My entire family does.

While those things are historical events now, they were just part of growing up for me. I remember going to a Baltimore Orioles game or a Washington Senators game just as much. I was 4- or 5-years old, and it was the first time I went to a major-league sporting event. I didn't want to watch the game, I wanted to run around under the bleachers, and that's what I did.

I remember being lonely in elementary school at Fort Meade. My Mom had enrolled me early, so I had started kindergarten on the Army base at the age of 4. I didn't really understand that I was one of the only Black kids in school, because the school at Ft. Meade was integrated.

I believe all schools on Army bases were. I was lonely because a lot of the kids wouldn't play with me. I didn't know why, but I believe now it was because I was Black.

Then there was that day in my first-grade classroom when the secretary came in and said that the President had been shot. At home, my mother had been watching "As the World Turns" on TV when the news broke. When I got home, she was trying to get in touch with her mother, my grandmother, in Texas. Communications around the country were difficult that day.

After we came home from Germany, with "home" meaning the United States, we lived in Fort Leonard Wood, Missouri, near Waynesville by the Lake of the Ozarks, not far from Kansas City. My oldest sister Beverly graduated from Waynesville High School.

When I was 9-years old, my brother Tony and I would take a cab from our home to the G.I. barracks, where we would shine shoes for the enlisted men there. I think it cost us a quarter to take a cab each way, and we would charge about 25 cents for a shine. They might give us a tip and it would be 35 or 40 cents. That's how we made our spending money, shining boots and shoes for a lot of enlisted men. When we were done, we'd take a cab home. We made $4 or $5 a day. For a kid that age, that was pretty good spending money.

We lived there less than a year before my father again was assigned to Fort Wolters, Texas, which is just west of the Dallas/Fort Worth metroplex. Fort Wolters is connected to Mineral Wells. Basically, my father requested to move back to where our home was.

Fort Wolters was a place where the Army trained its helicopter pilots, a vital mode of transportation and combat during the Vietnam War. A lot of U.S. Army pilots were trained there, and as far back as World War II, some German prisoners of war were kept at what was then called Camp Wolters. Some of those prisoners worked in Mineral Wells as part of a work-release program.

Right after we moved there, my parents built a brand new home. I believe it cost somewhere around $14,000. My parents had met another Black couple in Germany, a military couple with no kids. The husband was sent to Vietnam, and his wife didn't want to be alone, so she came and lived with us. She helped my mother keep house, because they had become close while we lived in Germany. Her name was Johnnie Mae.

I remember specifically on April 4, 1968, being awakened by a scream from Johnnie Mae. She had been shocked to find out that Dr. Martin Luther King Jr. had been assassinated the night before in Memphis. Then a few months later, Robert F Kennedy was assassinated. The country was shaken, and so were most connected to my family. I didn't notice so much the riots at the Democratic convention in Chicago in 1968, but while I was watching television I could see a lot of civil unrest in places like Los Angeles and Detroit.

I didn't pay much attention to politics during the summer of 1968, but I did know that the President of the United States was from Texas. I had come to realize that being a Texan, and even just living in Texas, meant having a tremendous amount of pride. Starting in elementary school, it was drilled into your head. Being a Texan was special, and that meant you were special.

From the fifth grade until I graduated high school, I don't really recall my family going through any financial hardship. My father had long before decided to join the military, and the U.S. Government did a tremendous job of providing security for us. We didn't have to worry about medical bills because we went to the military doctor.

Grocery bills were relatively low because even though we didn't live on the army base at Fort Wolters, we were able to buy groceries and goods where things were much more affordable. As I grew up, we never had many concerns that a lot of other Black families might have had. I felt fortunate that way, and certainly more secure.

So, I didn't grow up in poverty. We did pretty good, comparatively speaking. My parents were able to finance and build a brand new home. It was a nice home. I guess I would categorize myself as growing up in a military family rather than a Black family, even though we were both.

Growing up in a military family, my parents taught us that there were only four colors that mattered in life: the red, white and blue in the American flag, and Army green. Most of the time, while growing up in and around the military, from one family to another, there was a tremendous amount of equality. You would find much more acceptance of, and disregard for, color, in my opinion, in the military. These facts, both real and perceived, helped my self-esteem.

In the military there was so much equality. The military itself was the equalizer. We weren't just taught not to look at color; we were made to understand that color made no difference. In the military, especially when we lived in Germany on the Army base, we were just Americans.

I played sports on the base. When we split up teams, it was just "Who's the best?" or "Who's the fastest" or "Who can jump the highest?" That's how you divided up teams. I can't ever remember competition having anything to do with color.

When we returned to the States and eventually moved to Texas, the military still provided that buffer. Off the base, however, things were different, and much more obvious. There were some places I knew I couldn't go because of the color of my skin. I had people say to me, "You're a Black guy who wishes he was White. You just hang out with White people."

To me, I didn't just hang out with White people, I hung out with my friends. Some were Black, and some were White. I hung out with people I felt comfortable with. At the time, I didn't appreciate my ethnicity, or my heritage of being Black. I didn't want to be a "Black kid." I just wanted to be a kid. I didn't appreciate my Black-ness or my Black culture until years later. I never had to. It simply never really connected like that.

There were a lot of kids that I hung out with, including White kids who didn't have to be my friends. They easily could have said, "I can't." but they accepted me. These are men and women who I continue to be friends with, some by way of Facebook, people whom I have called my friends for years. They include guys I keep in touch with from junior high and high school. It might have been a lot easier for them if they didn't include me. They didn't have to invite me over to their homes, but they did. They were like me, they didn't care. Some were Black, some were White. Color didn't matter.

A lot of people will think that I was a fan of Muhammed Ali because I am a Black man and he was Black. Well, so was his main rival, Joe Frazier. My mother was a fan of Hank Aaron, and by extension so am I, but not because he's Black. Willie Mays is Black too. I'm probably not the typical Black kid who was born in the late 50s and spent most of his young life in Texas. The color of my skin is an identifier, but that's not who I am or who I was. I felt more comfortable with White kids because they didn't care that I am Black, while the Black kids wondered why I was hanging out with the White kids.

If I can sum it all up, I'd do it this way: being a kid in a military family in the late 50s and in the 60s provided an escape. I was able to escape the "poverty of the times," and I'm not talking just about economic poverty.

I didn't embrace the Black culture, because that would have been getting away from my norm. It would have been like someone embracing their White culture because it separates them from the rest of us. We—my brothers and sisters—all stayed in the middle. It took me a while to accept and embrace the culture of being Black.

One thing that did separate me from my other friends, was that during the 60s my father served two tours of duty in Vietnam, each tour lasting one year. During one tour he was stationed in Cam Ranh Bay. I knew that my father was in what I might call a "safe zone." He was never out on patrol, and he was never in the jungle. He was never involved in any combat. He was an engineer, assigned to help fix things that were broken.

He may have helped build a bridge or repair a truck or jeep or something like that, but he was never near any combat.

After he returned home, he told us a story about his domestic life in Vietnam. He had an apartment in Vietnam with another soldier. They would pay Vietnamese women to clean their apartments, cook and do other chores. It was all part of the culture there.

My father and his buddy were returning from work one day, and they saw a group of people surrounding what appeared to be a fight. They jumped out of the jeep to find out that these women had all been beating up on his cleaning lady. She had pierced ears and they had ripped her earlobe off. To me, as a kid, that was the purest evil that I'd ever heard. My father told me it was typical of the way people in Vietnam had to live and survive.

Compared to the suicide bombings we hear about today, or shootings at schools or the tragedy of 9/11, it doesn't compare on the scale of violence. That, however, was the level of fear that I had for my father while he was in Vietnam. We didn't get much past that. For some reason, I knew that he'd always return home safely.

Twice he was gone for a year. When you grow up in a stable environment as I did, and your father is gone for a year—and I know there is a lot worse that young people go through nowadays—that was almost unheard of. All my friends knew that my father was gone in Vietnam, and that I "didn't have a dad."

Of all the events that happened in the 1960s, the one that impacted me the most was the JFK assassination, because it happened in Dallas, Texas, which is just 60 miles or so from where I was born.

For years after the shooting, to get from Mineral Wells to my grandmother's house in Greenville, Texas, we'd drive through Dallas and go by the Texas School Book Depository. The Texas School Book Depository is where the shots were fired, and as we drove near it, it was always the topic of discussion.

There were eight kids in our station wagon (we only had one car), and we'd all look for it. Very seldom in the summer did we travel during the day because it was so hot. (I remember my mother saying,

"One day we're going to have a car with an air conditioner.")

We rode in that station wagon with no seatbelts, because at the time they weren't required by law. Inevitably, you'd hear someone say, "We're almost there." We did that dozens of times, and it's moments like that that helped cultivate my love and appreciation of history.

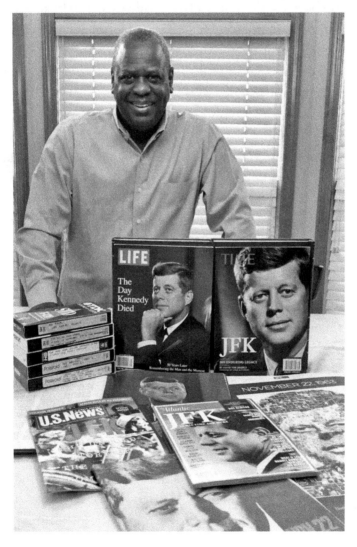

Al's affection for John F. Kennedy is well-known

In 1996, *The Kansas City Business Journal* found out that I collected hours and hours of documentaries and televisions specials on video tape, all dealing with the JFK assassination. The reporter called me at work. He said he had heard that I had a giant JFK video collection, and they wanted to interview me for a story.

I had collected 150 hours of JFK video tapes, which I still have. The History Channel was brand new at the time. That network was always airing special programming like that, so they aired hours and hours of programming connected to JFK. I recorded everything. I got material from other sources too, all on video tape.

Besides history, sports also played a noticeable role in my life as a kid growing up. Growing up in a family with four boys, sports were basically mandatory. My oldest brother Carlos is four years older than I am, then my next brother Anton, or Tony, is two years older and my younger brother Stephan is six years younger than I am. We were all involved with sports: basketball, baseball, football, even in Germany. When you weren't inside doing homework or chores, you played sports or games, and I mean all kinds of games.

If need be, we just went outside and played in the dirt. All you needed was a stick or a rock. We'd always make up some kind of game. Mostly though, we played ball. I was always a member of a sports team, in a sports league, be it Little League or Pony League or whatever.

When we moved to Texas, it got narrowed to football. If you grew up in Texas, that's what you did, because football was a year-round sport. As the old saying goes, there are three sports in Texas: football, politics and spring football.

Football was part of the fabric of who we were. When you grow up with that type of discipline, with a military father and a high school football coach, under the umbrella of the Church of Christ like I did, you had no excuses if you took the wrong path in life. You had the structure and you had the foundation. 'Nuff said.

As much as I enjoyed playing sports, I also enjoyed watching sports.

I always enjoyed watching Mickey Mantle, No. 7. There was only one baseball game a week on TV, on Saturday afternoon, the NBC Game of the Week. It seemed like the Yankees were always on.

On Sundays in the fall, the New York Giants and the New York Jets were always on. I had a big Joe Namath poster in my room. Most college football games weren't on TV, but on Sunday nights, I'd always watch the replay of a Notre Dame football game. Nowadays, you can watch 25 games on any given Saturday. That type of variety didn't exist in the 1960s and 70s. There was no ESPN or SEC Network or regional FOX Network.

I remember watching the Arkansas vs. Texas game in 1969. It was known as "The Game of the Century." No. 1 Texas fell behind No. 2 Arkansas 14-0 in Fayetteville in the fourth quarter, before winning 15-14 when James Street led the Longhorns on a late-game touchdown drive. Richard Nixon was the President of the United States. He visited the Texas locker room after the game.

I became infatuated with television, mainly from watching sports, and I always watched the news. More specifically, I always watched the sports segment on the news. My mother liked watching channel 8, WFAA, because Iola Johnson was the anchor and she was Black. In fact, she was the first Black female anchor in the Dallas/Ft. Worth market. My mother watched Iola Johnson and then years later she started watching Clarice Tinsley on KDFW, Channel 4, which was a CBS affiliate at the time.

As an aside, Clarice Tinsley is still anchoring there. She just celebrated her 40th year as a TV anchor. I was in TV for 40 years, and I thought that was quite an accomplishment. Clarice Tinsley worked on *one* anchor desk for 40 years.

When I was in Dallas in 2006 to cover Lamar Hunt's funeral, photographer Don Proctor and I had to go to KDFW to send some footage back to WDAF in Kansas City.

I was in the newsroom, waiting to feed tape, when Clarice Tinsley walked by and said, "Hey, who are you?" I told her I was from Kansas City and was there to cover Lamar Hunt's funeral. She said, "I'm Clarice Tinsley," and I said, "Oh, I know who you are." She seemed surprised.

I said, "My mother used to watch you every night, not to make you feel old, but right after she watched you, she watched *All In The Family* at 10:30." Clarice Tinsley then said, "Your mother watched me early in my career." I said, "Yes." Then she said, "How is she doing?" I said, "She passed away several years ago." She looked at me with such compassion. and then said, "Come here, give me a hug."

I hugged Clarice Tinsley. I was down there for Lamar Hunt's funeral, but to me that was the most compassionate moment of the whole 2½ days that Donnie and I were there.

My Mom got me hooked on Channel 8, which meant I watched Verne Lundquist every night doing sports. I just fell in love with television sports from the late 60s up until my senior year in high school, when I was faced with the decision, "What do you want to do with your life? What do you want to be?"

Since I was 12, I told people I wanted to be a sportscaster. I had to pick something to major in when I attended college. so why not pick that? I thought I'd give it a shot. I had no idea what was in front of me. I had no idea what the possibilities could be. I had no clue.

With all that transpired in the 1960s, both in our country and in my life, I've been asked often if there is one thing that impacted me the most. I can honestly say that it's not one single event. I think there are two things that connect my childhood and me working in television for 40 years. First of all, it would be the structure.

I find it very difficult to go from day to day without a foundation of structure, without a plan. That was a daily part of my life growing up. My friends wouldn't come over and knock on the door and say, "Can Alva come out and play?" They would knock on the door and say, "Has Alva done his chores?" Or they'd call and say, "Hey, man, are you done? Can you go? Are you done with all your stuff? Have you passed inspection?"

That's what my father called it when he'd check to see if we did our chores: "an inspection." He looked in drawers and made sure all the socks were in a row, and that kind of stuff. It wasn't a game with him; that's how he instilled his discipline in us. We had to empty trash cans around the house every day. I knew that even if I hadn't thrown any trash in that trash can since that time the day before, I still had to make sure it was empty.

My father would say, "Are you sure? Point being, if you're not sure and there's something in that trash can, then we're going to have words." When he really got mad at you, he wouldn't say, "I'm mad." He'd say, "I'm hot with you."

Back in those days, we didn't get spanked, we got a belt. After my father used the belt, he'd explain why he used it, and most often he'd say he loved us no matter what. So, the connection of my upbringing and working 40 years in television was structure.

The other connection was the sense of duty. In television we called it responsibility. You were responsible, especially when you got on the air, to the audience. You get a credential to a game. It doesn't matter if it's a high-school game or a college game or a professional game. That credential grants you a certain amount of access. After the game the coach is going to have a statement on why they won or lost or why they did what they did.

He can't have all 70,000 people at the Chiefs' game go into a postgame press conference. Only a select few get to do that. It was my responsibility as a member of the designated media, to get that information and pass it along to our audience.

There are a lot of things we all see happening in our lives every day. These events impact our lives, and we all need information about them, to help us live our lives and keep our communities and families safe. It's a reporter's responsibility to tell the public, and to do it truthfully, honestly and thoroughly.

Structure and responsibility. Those two things are connected. It wasn't one event, it was that sense of structure and responsibility that carried with me through 40 years. It helped lay that foundation. I was not only responsible to the public, I was responsible to everyone else in that newsroom, just like I was responsible to everyone in my family over the years, then and now. If I didn't do my job it made us all look bad.

CHAPTER 3

Darmstadt

DARMSTADT IS A fairly small town in south central Germany, 30 miles from Frankfurt. There was a U.S. Army base there established after World War II, closed down in 2008. It's not uncommon for there to be U.S. Army bases in various spots in Europe. A more famous one is in Wiesbaden, about 25 or 30 miles to the northwest of Darmstadt.

Thinking back over the last 15 or 20 years, you may have heard of someone from the United States who had been detained or held captive in the Middle East. When they are freed, they usually don't come straight to the United States. The government takes them to a military base somewhere in Europe for debriefing, to regroup or recuperate. Then, after all that, they return to the United States.

Quite often they would stop and stay in Wiesbaden. There's a large military hospital there. The American hostages, who were held captive in Iran and were finally released on the day President Ronald Reagan was inaugurated in 1981, first went to Wiesbaden when they were released.

My father was stationed at the base in Darmstadt from 1964 to 1967. With my parents and brothers and sisters, we were a family of ten. My oldest sister was 15 when we moved there, and my younger brother was just a year old. I was just shy of being seven years old.

There were dozens of military bases like Darmstadt and Wiesbaden, and they all had junior highs and high schools. A high school football team from one base would compete against the others, just like here in the United States, but on a different scale.

They also had semi-pro baseball teams. Some of the military guys would be on those teams. Life, to a large extent for a sports fan, was normal. Everybody was just affiliated with the military. The only difference was that we didn't go freely from one base to another. We were really secluded within our own community.

The main reason for the tight security at that time was the existence of East and West Germany. After World War II, the United States, Great Britain and France had recognized West Germany as a sovereign state. West Germany was three times the size of East Germany, but East Germany was the power and the threat to the U.S. It was scary, and as a kid, I always thought it represented something bad.

I have vivid memories of the threat of East Germany. I remember once, a friend and I were out riding bikes on the base. We had been told countless times: "Don't leave the base." but we were kids, so what did we do? We left the base.

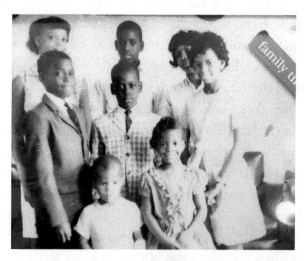

The three-year tour of duty in Germany brought the Wallace kids closer together

We barely got off the base, maybe by a block or two. Very quickly we saw one of those German motorcycles approaching with an attached sidecar. It looked like one of those motorcycles from the movie, *The Great Escape* starring Steve McQueen.

To me, they looked just like the German soldiers in that movie. They didn't have the Nazi insignias, but they were definitely German soldiers. Their uniforms, their helmets. their presence and their authority made me sweat bullets.

Those two soldiers were nice to us. They spoke poor, broken English, but they told us, "You shouldn't be here. Go back across the street." I remember the soldier in the sidecar. His leather boots came up to his knees. He was sitting back in that sidecar, and my eyes were drawn to one of his shiny boots, and my reflection in it. It was a scary sign of authority. They were telling us for our own protection, so we quickly went back. Every time I see a movie that has that type of costume or uniform, I think of that moment.

With all the freedoms we have in the United States, it's hard to imagine that ever-present threat. We were in the country of an ally, but there was still a feeling of uneasiness.

We were just barely two decades past World War II, so there were still some lingering tensions. East Germany was an ally of the Soviet Union. We were not friends with East Germany, and there was a wall in Berlin as evidence. We'd hear stories all the time about someone trying to escape from East Germany to the west, about somebody trying to build an armored car or use explosives to break through the wall.

As a kid, I listened to these stories, even though I knew some of them were romanticized and blown out of proportion. Some of the stories, however, were real. Every two months or so, there would be an air raid drill and we had to go to the basement of our apartment building in case we were being bombed or attacked.

There were three floors in our apartment complex, and we lived on the first level. On the fourth floor there was an empty attic. We could use that as a game room or use it as a party room. In one of the attics, you could see bullet holes in the wall.

They were real.

There was a lot of wooded area in Germany at the time, and it wasn't safe. Parents would say, "Don't go play in the woods." We'd hear about those who would walk in the woods and come across some type of unexploded grenade or other armament that was left from the war. It just wasn't safe.

The threat was not just against us because we were military. Living in Germany at the time meant you had to always be careful. As a kid, even more so. That was the reason for the protected area.

My oldest brother, Carlos once had a basketball game where he had to travel on a train. I don't know where they had to travel to, maybe Frankfort. He had to get on a train with his junior high basketball team. He remembers German soldiers getting on the train with machine guns. You didn't really hear about that often, but things like that happened.

The Army base provided a sense of security and protection. Even with that, we often felt we were living on an island. That sense also created a certain amount of unity. It simply brought everybody together. One family might be from Texas, another from California and a third family from the New England area. In Germany, we were all Americans. We had to stick together. That erased any racial or color barriers for the most part.

It was the great example of teamwork. It's like a professional team where one guy went to Michigan and another guy went to Ohio State, or one guy went to Duke and another guy went to North Carolina. It was cultural teamwork. The families were able to work past their differences because they had a greater common goal. That goal was to survive the two- or three-year tour of duty in Germany and return to the United States. The best way to do that was to stay together and be united.

Another thing to keep in mind was the fact that the Army base at Darmstadt was very American in a lot of ways, not the least of which were the sports that we played. Soccer may have been huge in Germany at the time, but you would have never known it on our Army base. We played sports that were popular in America. I don't remember soccer at all. This was an American base, not a European base. Soccer wasn't big in the United States, and we just weren't exposed to it. German soldiers and citizens generally weren't allowed on the base.

We knew the people who lived in the town were German. There was no real interaction that I knew of between American families and German families. Nothing between German soldiers and American families. They weren't allowed on the base, and we weren't really allowed off the base without supervision. It was an island. If there was any resentment of Americans by the Germans because of World War II, I never heard about it.

Even though we lived on an American Army base, we were able to experience several aspects of the German culture. When I was 8 or 9 years old, I could speak German almost as well as I could speak English. I learned the German language, ate German food, even wore some German clothes—like lederhosen. Every Friday a beer truck would come by and sell German beer in the neighborhood. My parents often would buy a couple of bottles of beer, and the bottles were huge. So we were exposed to German culture.

While living in Darmstadt, I experienced the first time someone would point out to me that I was different, and not accepted, because of my skin color. The news had circulated at school that there was a Cub Scout den being started, and a lot of my friends and I were excited to join. We all lived in these huge apartment complexes on the Army base. The buildings all had numbers. My family lived in Building 4411, apartment C2. This Cub Scout meeting was being held at another building about five minutes away, and the den mother was the mom of a kid at my school.

I went to the first Cub Scout meeting, and the den mother came to me and said, "You don't belong here, you're in the wrong den. You're not supposed to be here." She showed me some piece of paper, some application that I had brought, she said, "See, you're over here in 4411. You're supposed to be somewhere else." So, 15 minutes after I had left home, I was back. I walked in the door and my mother said, "What happened? I thought you had a Cub Scout meeting?" I told her that the den mother said that I was in the wrong place.

My mother looked at the application and said, "She's just prejudiced. She just didn't want you there." She used the word "prejudiced." I said, "What's that?" My mother replied, "Don't worry about it. We'll get you in another den." The next week I was in another den and all was well. My mother had used that word—prejudice. She could have gone into the whole explanation, but she just said, "Don't worry about it." I remember it like it was yesterday.

It was less than 10 years after we moved back from Germany to the United States that I was a student at Texas Tech. I was away from Germany for 11 years when I got my first job in television. It was only 14 years after Germany that I was named sports director at KAMC in Lubbock. I mention the time frames because life is all about perspective, and it all goes by so fast.

I've been asked if I ever had the desire to blend the two, to cover a sporting event in Germany or anywhere in Europe, and the answer would be no. I've never covered a sporting event on foreign soil, other than covering Royals postseason baseball in Toronto. I would have loved to, but not at the expense of my true love in sports journalism, like covering NCAA and Kansas basketball in March.

Living in Germany for those three years provided some valuable life lessons, not just for me, but for our entire family. Having to live out of our comfort zone of the United States made us bond together and stay together. It also made us realize that we shouldn't take anything for granted. The freedoms that we are allowed in the United States really don't exist anywhere else in the world. The opportunities that we are allowed in this country, don't really exist anywhere else in the world. Those freedoms and opportunities are precious, and my entire family would again be exposed to them when we moved back to the United States in 1967.

CHAPTER 4

One for the Coyotes

IF YOU EVER win the lottery, and you've got millions of dollars to burn, may I suggest you rent a Learjet. On a clear, October Friday evening, fly as low as you can across the state of Texas. No doubt you'll notice all the lights from the stadiums that are hosting high school football games. You can do that in any state in the country, but you'll see more in Texas, and you'll never cover the entire state.

I did something similar once, though not in a Learjet, and I saw nowhere near the entire state. I flew on the team charter with the Texas Tech football team when they played in Arkansas. We flew from Lubbock to Little Rock, Arkansas. Flying across the state of Texas, I saw a lot of football stadiums. I thought that trip was majestic.

As the old saying goes—and as I said before—there are three sports in Texas: football, politics and spring football. In Texas, football permeates your life. It permeates your culture, it is among the most important pieces of structure that I can think of that helped me become the person I am. The sport of football in Texas consumes you. It has a significant amount of importance to each and every community, big or small, rich or poor, Black or White.

Texas high school football transcends racial barriers. It's a 12-month-a-year existence. Texans feels it's unique. Texas is still the only state that can split up into five different states, a unique condition to the annexation to the Union in 1845. State pride is part of the foundation of your education during grades 1-12. In the state of Texas educational system, state history takes precedence over American history. American history is important, but growing up I always felt it wasn't as important to Texans as Texas history.

Football is a big part of that. From the team to the coaches to the school to the cheerleaders to the parents to the booster club, it's all part of the economic engine that drives each and every community.

I grew up with that mindset from the fifth grade until I graduated from high school and enrolled at Texas Tech. The importance of Texas high school football was drilled into me, along with the structure and the discipline that it provides.

From the time I was in seventh grade through my junior year, the head coach of Mineral Wells High School was a man named Frank Beavers. It's like if you're from Kansas City and you say, "I played under Tony Severino," chances are good that you played at Rockhurst High School.

During my junior year at Mineral Wells High School with Frank Beavers at head coach, I had a teammate, a running back named Alvin Garrett. Alvin was part of the group of receivers that later was called the "Fun Bunch," and helped the Washington Redskins beat the Miami Dolphins in Super Bowl XVII.

Frank Beavers once challenged the team by saying, "Name one other activity, *other than church*, where young people can meet once a week, for the good of the community, and have something positive come out of it." I've searched high and low, and I can't think of another thing.

Right after my junior year of high school, Coach Beavers left Mineral Wells and took a job at Highland Park High School in Dallas. Highland Park High School produced NFL quarterback Matthew Stafford, and MLB pitcher Clayton Kershaw. I know Highland Park more for producing quarterback Lance McIlhenny and offensive lineman David Richards, who both went on to play at SMU. Highland Park High School is among the best resourced school districts in the biggest class in the state.

One thing that is fairly unique about Texas high school football is that the same offensive and defensive schemes are played at every level of football in most school districts. In Texas, it dates back to the 1960s, while that concept only hit the Kansas City area in the last 20 or 30 years.

Coaching staffs would teach one offense and one defense to the sixth and seventh graders. By the time they were in high school, they'd been in the system for a while and were able to execute it better because they knew it better. When you were in junior high in Mineral Wells—there were three junior high schools—they all ran the Houston Veer offense designed by the legendary Bill Yeoman, who coached for years at the University of Houston.

While I was growing up in Mineral Wells, football teams didn't run the wishbone or the power-I. We ran the Houston Veer in seventh, eighth and ninth grade. When you got to high school, you already had the experience. Everything about the offense had become second nature.

As head coach at the high school, Coach Beavers installed that system into all the football programs in Mineral Wells. He was also a strict disciplinarian. Our regular season schedule was done by the third weekend of November, so we started our off-season program during the month of December.

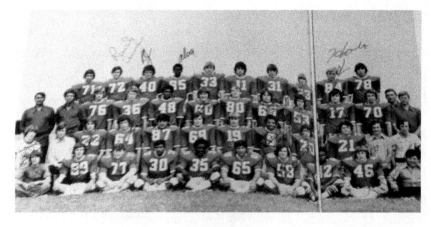

Al wore No. 85 on the 1974 Mineral Wells High School Rams

After the Christmas holidays, we started our weight program. Spring football hit in late March or April, with three weeks in full pads on the field. Our weight program after school consisted of 30 minutes of weights, 30 minutes of agility drills and 30 minutes of cardio. During the spring, we were at school until 5 p.m. or later.

With the weight drills and agility drills, we did three sets of 10 at each station—bench press, jump rope or climbing rope, to name a few. Coach Beavers was an excellent motivator, and though I don't remember him saying it out loud, we knew he truly believed, "To be the best you, you've got to beat the best."

The best high school football program in Texas in the late-60s through the mid-70s was Wichita Falls High School, the Wichita Falls "Coyotes." They had won six state championships through the years.

Wichita Falls High had a quarterback named Ronnie Littleton who later went to play at TCU. Rumor had it that TCU gave him a car. To a kid from Mineral Wells, that seemed unimaginable. NCAA rules at the time weren't as stringent as they are today. The University of Texas had a lot of success in part because they were good, and in part because scholarship limits were much different than they are now.

The Wichita Falls School District had a stadium with artificial turf, and that was in the early 70s. They might as well have been a college program. They were the "best of the best" in Texas.

Coach Beavers said, "If you're going to beat those guys, then you've got to do a little more, you've got to work a little harder." When you finished your stations with the 10 weight repetitions, he'd always suggest doing one more. Instead of 10, do 11. Do "One for the Coyotes."

He may have been talking about football, but that attitude could benefit you for the rest of your life too. If you want to be the best that you can be throughout your daily work, throughout your daily life, you've got to do what is expected, but you've also got to do just a little bit more, or "One for the Coyotes." You've got to be just a little bit better, and work just a little bit harder, to be the best.

"One for the Coyotes." That's the work ethic I used throughout my 40 years in broadcasting, and throughout life in general. Even today, I'll go to the gym with my wife. We'll walk the track for 30 minutes, and I'll say, "One for the Coyotes," and she'll say, "Okay," and we'll walk the track for another minute or another lap.

I mentioned something earlier in passing that I believe needs to be emphasized. When I say, "Texas high school football," I'm not just saying high school football that's played in Texas. "Texas high school football" is an entity in and of itself. It's different from high school football in any other state, because of the importance in the community. There's an element of pride and ownership involved.

It's not gumbo, it's Louisiana gumbo. It's not bar-b-que, it's Kansas City bar-b-que. It's different from football, it's different from high school football. To me, it's "Texas high school football," because, in my opinion, it's better. It's separate, and not equal.

While playing high school football, I was a wide receiver and defensive back, and I was one of three team captains. I understood the importance of football, but I didn't understand the importance of education. I didn't understand the importance of going to class, paying attention and making good grades.

My grades were good enough to get into Texas Tech, but they weren't good enough to get into TCU or Texas. I'd always dreamed of playing at Tennessee because I wanted to be Condredge Holloway, the former Tennessee Volunteer quarterback.

When I was in seventh grade, I attended Austin Junior High. For some reason we were the Orange Volunteers. We had bright orange jerseys. I loved Condredge Holloway, but I couldn't even dream of being good enough to play at Tennessee.

I still wanted to play college football. If I couldn't play at Tennessee, I wanted to play football in the Southwest Conference. I did walk on for two weeks at Texas Tech before I got cut from the roster. I thought I was good enough to play Southwest Conference football, and for two weeks I was, but only in practice.

As far as an education, Texas Tech was exactly my speed. It was far enough away from home that I couldn't come home every day, but if I had to get home for an emergency, I could. It was about a four-and-a-half-hour drive.

I figured going to school at Tech would be like high school, and starting out, I can honestly say I didn't really have a real academic plan. I didn't realize it at all until football season was over in November 1974, and I was going to graduate in May 1975. The most important thing in my life—Texas high school football—was over. I didn't understand. It took me about three years and three months of college until I found something that was as good, as important, as football. It took that long.

It might surprise you, considering all I've told you about structure from my parents and the military, that I took the easy way out. I wasn't lazy. I just didn't know what I didn't know. I didn't care. Also, I didn't listen. I didn't understand. Mineral Wells is about the size of Leavenworth, Kan. I was good in sports there. I was good in football. I figured that was enough.

I soon found out that I wasn't good enough to play football at Tech, and my "just get by" attitude wasn't going to cut it in the classroom. I'm not sure why, but I didn't apply "One for the Coyotes" to my education. When I got to college, my grades were just good enough to stay in school. I made some failing grades in college. I had to take a class or two over. I definitely wasn't on a four-year path to graduate.

It wasn't until the summer of 1978 that I reached the point that I had to change. After three years there, I was barely classified as a junior because of bad grades. I went home for the summer of 1978, I messed around and didn't save a nickel. I may have saved $500, but back then the whole school year may have cost $3,000 or $4,000. My parents had made it obvious they weren't going to pay for my continuing education.

When it was time to go back to school. my Dad said, "You've saved no money. You've done nothing to get ready to go back to school." The morning I left, he bought me a tank of gas, gave me a $5 bill and said, "I'll see you in two weeks." He thought if I couldn't find a job and I couldn't go to school, he'd see me in two weeks.

That was my incentive to do something. So as soon as I got to Lubbock in late August, I got a job parking cars. I was doing something and making some money. My parents had always told us if we found a job, whatever we'd make, they'd help us and try to match half of that.

I hated parking cars. I had to go to downtown Lubbock, and I had to get up at 5 or 5:30 to be at work at 6 a.m. All the business people would come to town, and I'd park their cars. Class hadn't started yet, but that got old really quickly.

I also applied for a job at the *Lubbock Avalanche-Journal*, the local newspaper. That job required me to be at work at midnight to take the freshly printed newspapers off the printer. I quit the job parking cars, and I accepted the job at the *Avalanche-Journal*, where part of the job description had me skeptical.

I would have to get some of those white tube socks, the ones that come up to your knees. I was supposed to put the tube socks on my arms, so when the newspaper came off the printer, I wouldn't get ink all over my hands and arms. That sounded like no fun at all, a great big mess.

Getting ready for the fall semester of 1978, I shared an apartment with two roommates. The Sunday before Labor Day—I was supposed to start at the newspaper that night and there was no school on Monday—we had about 15 to 20 people over to our apartment for a party. We had burgers and beer. Everybody partied, but I wasn't drinking because I had to be at work at midnight. People were asking, "You've got to go to work? Really? What's up with you?" That lasted throughout the evening.

At about 11:30 p.m., I said to myself, "I can't do this job," and I just decided not to show up. That was as bad a thing as I've ever done in committing to do a job and not showing up for that job. I also did a bad thing by not working hard that summer, which allowed my dilemma to continue, I needed to find a part-time job to support myself.

I had a friend at Tech who was from Fort Worth. She had just finished her freshman year. She stayed in Lubbock that summer and lived with her older sister. She had gotten a job at KAMC, the ABC TV station. I asked her, "How did you do that?" She said, "I just went in and asked. I heard they had an opening and I went in and applied. I sweep the floor and run teleprompter for the newscast."

That friend was at that pre-Labor Day party. She said, "You ought to apply there." I went there a day or two later and applied for a job. On September 8, 1978, right after Labor Day, I landed my first job in television. I was working in the production department, sweeping floors and running prompter for the newscast. I made $2.90/hour.

While "One for the Coyotes" probably didn't apply to my education, or my dedication to finding work in the fall of 1978, another theory that I've used often in my career did. I call it the "Head Cheerleader Syndrome." It fits perfectly on how I got that first job at KAMC.

The stereotypical description of the head cheerleader in high school is the best-looking gal in school. She makes great grades and she dates the football captain. This *imaginary* head cheerleader, however, doesn't date anyone. She's the head cheerleader and she makes great grades. She's got all those credentials, but she doesn't have a boyfriend. Why not? Because nobody believes she's going to say "yes" if they ask her out.

They believe she's too good for them, so she goes every Saturday night without a date. The football game is Friday night, so she can't have a date that night. Every Saturday night she sits at home without a date because no one will ask her out.

My question to all those guys out there who don't think she'll go out with them is, "Why not you? What's the worst that's going to happen to you if you ask her out? She says 'no'? Is she going to call the police, and say, 'This guy asked me out, arrest him? He's a threat to national security.'" I truly believe she wouldn't say any of that. The worst thing she'd say is "no." There's also a chance she'd say "yes."

Most guys don't ask her out because they're afraid she's going to say "no," because they've elevated her above the standard they think of themselves. They don't see themselves as worthy. It's a vicious circle. She doesn't go out because no one will ask her. They don't ask because they don't think she will say "yes." I say, "Get off your butt and ask her out," or "Get off your butt and go ask for the job."

Over the years at WDAF in Kansas City, I had a lot of young people apply for internships. They would come in in a suit and tie with a resume. They're all ready. I noticed that, but it never really mattered to me. The dynamics that I felt were important went beyond what was on the resume. They were things that were more personal and practical. What kind of effort and work ethic did they possess? Were they willing to ask the head cheerleader for a date? Were they willing to work hard to get and keep the job?

I can't say I was always perfect. Remember, I'm the guy who rode the media elevator 10 times, just to interact with Marlena. It took me a while to ask her where a guy could meet her away from campus.

One question I would ask an interviewing intern is, "What makes you think you can't get this internship?" They'd say, "Well, this is WDAF." I'd tell them We are all human, just like you. If you're a student at JUCO or K-State or Mizzou or KU or whatever, if you qualify and there's an opening and you handle everything right, you might get the job. The worst we're going to do is say "no."

The internship is there to provide an opportunity. Often, we only had one candidate. There were some summers where we had three interns. That line of logic has always stuck with me (I guess with the exception of falling in love). When I went to the locker room after a game, some reporters are afraid to ask questions of the big star. The worst he's going to do is say "no." Sometimes they say, "I don't want to talk."

That's their bad, not my bad or an intern's bad. I didn't have a problem going up and talking to people, as long as I did it properly. So that "head cheerleader syndrome," although I didn't realize it at the time, was what got me my first job at KAMC. I went and asked for a job I didn't think I was qualified for, but absolutely I was.

It was just sweeping the floors and running a teleprompter for $2.90/hour, but I was working in television. There was a lot of turnover in that job, but when I got it, I wanted to hang onto it. I could tell after a couple of days, certainly a couple of weeks, that I loved it.

KAMC recorded and aired the "Rex Dockery Show." He had just been hired as head coach at Texas Tech. After the show was recorded, someone would have to take the tape reel to the airport, so it could be flown to and air at other stations across the state, in markets like Dallas/Ft. Worth, Houston and San Antonio. It aired in Dallas on KTVT, Channel 11. My parents could watch that station at our home in Mineral Wells.

The first show that I knew had my name on the credits was later in the fall. Near the end of the show, when I knew the credits were rolling and I knew that my parents were watching, I called home. I heard my Mom in the background, "There he is!" For the first time ever, they saw my name on TV.

That to me was just like covering the Royals when they won the World Series. When my parents saw my name on the credits, it was a validation that yes, I did have a job at a TV station.

All because I ignored the "head cheerleader syndrome."

I guess I had been lazy. I had been lazy in the classroom, I'd been lazy that previous summer. I had played Texas high school football, and I thought that was enough. I didn't have to do anything else. I was resting on the laurels that I thought I had, but actually didn't. That time in my life was all over.

During the month of September 1978, I began to realize my professional life truly did have a purpose.

CHAPTER 5

Woody and KAMC

YOU NEVER KNOW what people you will meet throughout your life who will have a long-lasting impact on your life. John "Woody" Curry had a huge impact on my life in a number of ways.

During the late summer of 1978, I had no desire to build my career around parking cars. I also figured out, before my first day on the job, that I didn't want to work midnights, so I never went to work at the *Lubbock Avalanche-Journal*. What turned out to be my career for more than 40 years was not as much orchestrated as it was happenstance.

I mentioned that a friend at Texas Tech suggested that I apply for a job at the local ABC affiliate—KAMC—because they were hiring. I was majoring in telecommunications, so maybe it would look good on my resume.

Why would they hire me, a guy barely keeping his head above water from a grade standpoint? Who knows? I figured it was worth challenging the "head cheerleader syndrome" and at least apply.

Everybody called KAMC, "K-Mac" because the station owner was a man named Bill McAlister. Bill and his father started the station back in the 1950s. Lubbock, Texas, is the hometown of the late Buddy Holly. The McAlisters also owned a radio station, KSEL. Before Buddy

Holly became nationally known as a rock and roll singer, he would play around Lubbock in a lot of different places. He would play at sock-hops, at the bowling alley and the Dairy Queen.

The McAlister family would have him in their studio and on the radio station. When I got my job at KAMC almost 20 years after Buddy Holly died, Bill McAllister was also the mayor of Lubbock. So it was a very well-known family.

Among the staff of news reporters at KAMC in 1978 was a reporter by the name of Scott Pelley. Scott later moved to jobs in TV news in Dallas, and then to New York as the anchor for CBS News and 60 Minutes. During my very early years at KAMC, I always got a kick out of Scott entering the studio with no shoes on. He would run and 'slide' the last six feet or so to the set in his socks with no shoes on.

I applied for a job in the production department. Woody was the production manager, so he was the guy who hired me. I filled out the application and sat in his office for an interview for about 10 or 15 minutes. He said, "Okay, we'll give you a call, and let you know one way or another."

Within an hour or so, he called and said, "This job is yours if you want it. You'll start at $2.90 an hour. You'll work in production. I can only give you 20 hours a week right now." I jumped on it. That started my 40 years in broadcasting, September 8, 1978, at a small TV station that employed about 40 people.

I could tell almost immediately that Woody personified a lot of things that I valued: structure, infrastructure, dedication and responsibility. Along with all of that, Woody was the kind of guy who liked to have a good time. He preferred an atmosphere that included having fun on the job. You could talk to him. He spoke plain English; he was very understandable when he communicated, though he could also use technical terms too.

I learned very quickly that television production could be a lot like football. The boss, or the "coach," could love you up and he could love

45

you down. Woody always told me, "When you're doing a newscast and you're on headsets, just because you do something wrong between 6:00 and 6:28 during the newscast, and I get unhappy with you over headsets, it doesn't mean that I don't like you. I just don't like what you did." Woody taught me that in the heat and pressure of television, it's best not to take criticism personally.

A football coach might not like the way a player had bad form on a tackle, catching a pass or throwing a pass, or the way he lined up, he probably still likes him. Most parents say at one point or another, "You made a mistake and I yelled at you. It doesn't mean that I don't love you or like you. I just don't like what you did."

Looking back over my life, I realize now that Woody was a great leader, a role model and someone I wanted to learn from. He was so well respected.

It wasn't until years later, after not seeing him for more than 10 years, that I found out that he had died of cancer. I got the news of his passing while having a casual conversation with another guy who used to work for Woody. I said, "How's Woody?" He said, hesitantly, "Woody died last year. He had cancer." I just sat there, silent and stunned. I eventually teared up. I couldn't believe it. I couldn't believe that I had become that disconnected from him.

I learned so much from him, because he knew how to relate to different people. Woody knew how to talk to me as a young Black man. He knew how to talk to another person who had grown up in a much different environment than mine. He could talk to the entire spectrum of his staff. We were all from different socioeconomic backgrounds and lives.

In TV, when you're part of the newscast or part of the production crew, you're all one. You're all part of the team. I knew that working in television involved a lot of teamwork, from the beginning to the end of the day, and to be even more specific, from the beginning to the end of a newscast.

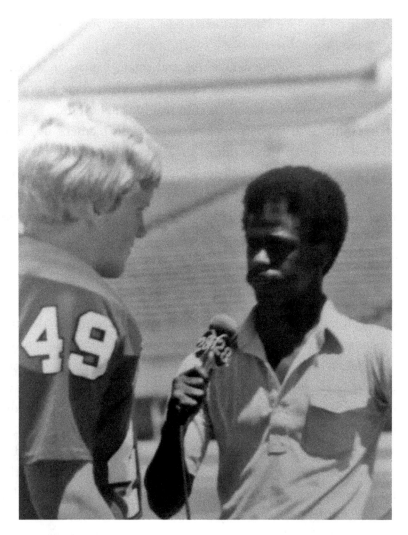

The Texas Tech Red Raiders, including linebacker Jeff McKinney,
were Al's first taste of big-time college football.

One of the things that I appreciated most about Woody was that
he may have hired me for an entry-level position, but he didn't treat
me as an entry-level employee. He trained me as if I was a person who
was going to be in television broadcasting or sports broadcasting for 40
years, and he took that approach with everyone.

47

It wasn't like, "We have an extra position and you get to push a broom." He invested in me like a coach invests in a player. He taught me the importance of the details, big and small. I mentioned earlier about my love of history and my belief that in life, there is nothing insignificant. Woody taught me that in real-life application.

For example, a cable connected to a studio camera might be considered an insignificant thing. In a television studio, there are numerous cables coming out of the wall, connected to cameras. These cables were 25 or 30 feet long, and the cameras were on pedestals that you rolled around the studio. The more tension you put on the cables, or the more you bend or use and abuse them over the years, the more the cables become weakened.

When you stored those cables, you had to do it the right way. You didn't just leave the cables strung out over the floor, because that was an opportunity for something to roll over it or someone to walk on it, and it endangers that cable. So we rolled the cables up a certain way.

My father used to say, "If you take care of your car, it will take care of you." He meant that if you needed to go somewhere, the car would have to be operational. If you didn't take care of it, it wouldn't be operational when you needed it.

That's the way Woody treated equipment in the studio and in the control room. Production personnel needed to take care of that equipment, because we were going to need it to work. Little things like that made a difference to Woody, and he made sure we knew it.

There was a lot of turnover in the production department, because the pay wasn't great, and neither were the hours. On weekends when I started, I'd work on Saturdays from 9 a.m. to 1 p.m., then again later that day from 8 p.m. to 11.p.m. The days and hours were fractured. I'd have to work nights, often when my college roommates and other friends were out having a good time. A lot of people would work in production at KAMC for three or four months, or even three or four weeks, and then say, "I got another job paying me $3.20/hour. I've got to go."

For some reason, I stuck with it. I loved working in television. I liked the structure, I liked the specialness of working in television. Nobody I knew had done this before. I knew it was different and I felt it was special. I thought, "Maybe this can lead to something. Maybe this can lead to me working in television sports." That, at least, was the hope and goal.

Woody was a big part, certainly initially, of that reasoning. At the time he was a single guy, at times working 10-hour days. He had to manage his staff, and he had to answer to the general manager. Woody was part of a staff of department heads, and they all answered to Bill McAlister.

I'm not sure he was really aware of it, but he wound up teaching me a lot. Even though I'd been in school for three years, I learned more in that first month at KAMC than I had learned in three years of college. The job was all hands-on. It was all real.

A television studio and control room weren't like a classroom or something to make a good grade on with a test. I didn't like school, but I did like my job, a lot. Maybe Woody saw that I liked it too.

We had a conversation during my first two weeks of working there. He told me, "You'll do this for two weeks and you'll know whether this is what you want to do for the rest of your life." He was right, and over the years I would think about that often.

I think what really captured my heart was that fact that it was "live" television, and its success or failure had consequences. You couldn't screw it up. There are no do-overs in live television. The most important obligation for a local TV station is to deliver the news. The most important revenue-maker for a local television station is its local newscast. The newscast gives the station its local identity. The newscast is where it most often sells its most valuable commercials. The news department and news presentation is its most important connection and service to the local community.

Being a part of a live newscast was like being in a game. We aired a 6 p.m. and 10 p.m. newscasts, five nights a week. To me, that was like playing in two games a day. (On weekends, we only aired a 10 p.m. newscast.) For me, a guy who enjoyed playing high school football, it was great to have two games a day. That game only lasted 30 minutes, but it took all day to get ready for that 24-minute game (when you factor in the commercial breaks). It was a big-time adrenalin rush, that required preparation, dedication, responsibility and execution.

I spent about six and a half years at KAMC, and not all of that time was working under Woody. Woody had married Pam Baird, and she became news director in early 1981. She eventually appointed me sports director at KAMC on September 8, 1981, three years to the day after I was first hired at the station.

I followed a fairly normal progression of job responsibility in the production department at KAMC, but it wasn't always a smooth path. There are numerous jobs and tasks involved that go into putting a television newscast on the air. To me, it was just like being on a football team. You have the guys on the roster and the coaches, plus the equipment people: the trainers, all the people who help the team get ready for the game.

The natural order of ascent in the production department at KAMC was to work in the studio, to learn to operate the cameras and learn what camera angles work best. You'd learn how to work in the studio before you got a promotion—and a raise of $.20 an hour or so—to the control room.

In the KAMC control room, the first thing you did was work the film chain. The film chain was a contraption that was about four-inches thick and 12-inches round, almost like the hub of a wheel. The film chain operator was in charge of putting different slides into the film chain throughout the newscast to provide the graphic behind the on-air person. If it was upside down in the film chain, it was right side up on the air.

The next step in job progression was videotape operator, which was more complicated. The all-important commercials aired from videotape, and a lot of news stories aired from videotape too. After working with the videotape machines, the next job on the ladder of job responsibility was operating the audio board, and after that, the video switcher. The video switcher is operated by the technical director, who punches up each video source that eventually winds up on air.

Finally, you had a director, who was in charge of all the production personnel working within the newscast. The director called all the shots. The director had the final say before and during a newscast, and any commercial production that we did.

In a year and a half, I had worked my way up to audio, and my next progression was to be a technical director. I loved TV production. I loved making TV, but I also had another opportunity that presented itself in the news department.

The sports anchor was Doug Rains. Doug and I talked quite often during commercial breaks of the newscast, and throughout the day during down time. He'd say, "Did you see the game last night?" or "What did you think about that coaching decision?" He knew that I had a high interest in sports, so occasionally he would invite me back to the sports office to assist in some way, like ripping wire copy or helping him collect scores. I'd hang out in the sports office when I had time.

That led to an opportunity to begin an internship in sports. I would get college credit for it. Sometimes I'd be walking down the hall at KAMC and someone would say to me, "Hey, you're not working today. What are you doing here?" And I'd say, "I'm interning in sports." It got to the point many times where I was spending seven days a week at the television station.

Before I knew it, I was spending the majority of my time in the sports department. By late 1980, station management asked me if I wanted to work 20 hours in sports and 20 hours in production and get paid for both. I was able to make the transition and it became apparent—to some I guess—that I had some talent.

Pam Baird was only a few years older than I was. After my internship, I began anchoring sports on the weekends, even though I was still in school. I think I was doing an okay job, but not according to Pam. More than once she told me I was the biggest screw-up. She had given me this job as weekend anchor, and I couldn't do anything right. This went on for a couple of months. She kept pulling me into her office and ripping me up and down.

I wasn't ready to quit, but certainly I was struggling with the perception that I couldn't do anything right.

In late August 1981, she pulled me into her office again. I just figured she was getting ready to rip me another one. However, to my surprise, she said, "I've been hard on you. One reason why is because I see a lot of promise in you. What I want to do is fire Doug and make you sports director." I was floored. Then she added, "And I want to do it next week."

So, on September 8, 1981, three years to the day after I was hired, I became sports director at KAMC in Lubbock, Texas.

What was difficult about the transition to sports director was that we had two sports anchors. I did weekends and Doug anchored weeknights. When I became the main guy, we didn't have a weekend guy. So, for about six weeks, I worked every day, seven days a week, while we searched for a weekend anchor.

This may have been my first professional application of "One for the Coyotes." I'm not saying I didn't show concern about it, but I don't remember complaining. I had to do what I had to do. Sometimes in a game you're tired, you're about to break down, but you have to keep playing.

I did the extra little things, the repetitions, the extra work in this case, the extra two shifts, to do what needed to be done. I wanted to be the best sports director I could be, and if it didn't work out, it wouldn't be because I didn't work hard.

Eventually we hired a weekend sports anchor named Bill Jones. Bill had been in law school at the University of Oklahoma, after having grown up in Irving, Texas, where his father was an attorney. He had attended Irving MacArthur High School, the same high school that produced Oklahoma linebacking great Brian Bosworth.

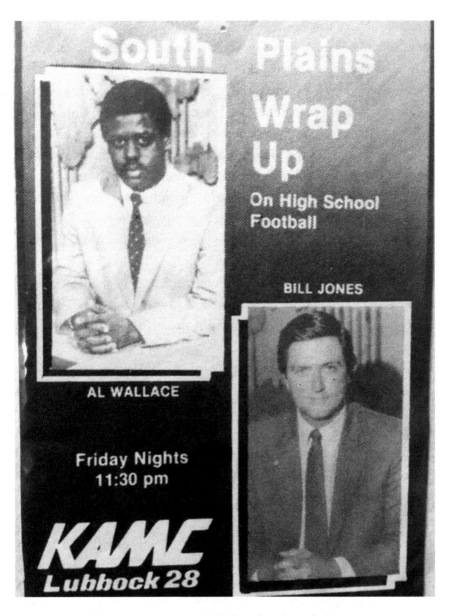

South Plains Wrap Up

On High School Football

BILL JONES

AL WALLACE

Friday Nights
11:30 pm

KAMC
Lubbock 28

Bill Jones remains one of Al's best friends in the business

Pam Baird had attended Irving MacArthur and knew Bill's older sister. Pam was talking with his sister, and she told Pam that Bill was looking for a sports job in television. We both looked at his audition tape and we loved it. Two weeks later Bill came to Lubbock, and almost immediately he decided to join the staff. To this day, he's one of the best friends I've ever had in TV. His broadcast career has eclipsed mine, and not just in market size. He knows Dallas-Ft. Worth sports history better than anyone I've ever known.

Kansas City has the Simone Award for the best area high school football player. In Dallas, they have the Tom Landry Award, and Bill presents that award every year. I worked with him for three and a half years, and later would be a groomsman in his wedding.

Eventually, I wound up at a point where nine plus years in Lubbock were enough. I knew I needed to move on. KAMC, like a lot of stations at that time, worked with a consulting company. The company would advise the station on things like how the anchors should dress, what the weather guy should do, etc. They would also help the station develop a news theme and with marketing.

KAMC had consulting company for several years called Audience Research and Development— or ARD. Somewhere along the line, that company and the station ran afoul. There was a separation. Shortly after that, I got a call from ARD, telling me that they had been hired by a competing station in Lubbock. The guy explained that they had divorced KAMC because they had given the station advice and station management refused to take it.

He said, "We're working for Channel 11, KCBD, the NBC affiliate. They feel like you are a pain in their (rear), and they want to get rid of you. We want to help you find a job in another market."

I was looking to leave, so I said, "If you can help me find a job, I'm listening." ARD told me they had a station in Las Vegas that was looking for someone just like me. The next day the news director from the station in Las Vegas called me. Forty-eight hours earlier, Las Vegas was the last place in the world I wanted to work or live. But my desire to leave West Texas outweighed just about every other option.

It was a compliment that the other station wanted me to leave town. It's like one school that wants to beat another school in college football. They'll say, "Let's get rid of the coach that always wins the league title by getting another school in another league to hire him." To me, that would be a compliment. I look back on that time and feel pretty good about it.

Taking the job in Las Vegas seemed like an easy decision, but it was more complicated than that. At the time, my younger brother Stephan was an undergrad at Texas Tech. When I got the call from Las Vegas, we were living together. After I got the call, I told him that I had a chance to leave. I didn't want to leave him in a lurch. Stephan said, "Don't worry about me. I'll be fine. If you need to go, go." So the decision was made.

A week later, the station in Las Vegas flew me out for an interview and offered me the job. It only took a couple of days for me to accept it. Three weeks later, I was working in Las Vegas, Nevada. It would be a complete change in climate, personal life, professional life and in every other way.

CHAPTER 6

Vegas, Baby

LAS VEGAS, NEV., is the only place in the country where you can go to a grocery store and play a slot machine. I'd say that's a whole lot different than Lubbock, Texas. From the moment I accepted the opportunity to interview for the job in Las Vegas, things in my life were a bit off-center and would require a noticeable amount of adjustment.

In the end, I would live in Las Vegas for only three months. I would later realize those 90 days were necessary for me to become the person I am today. During that three-month detour, I learned that nothing is guaranteed. I felt like I had "done 10 years" in Lubbock, but I also had to "do three months" in Vegas.

Las Vegas was a massive curve ball. It was a pitch in the dirt, and I went for it. I eventually got on base, but then I had to figure out how I was going to "get home." In the end, I'm not sure Kansas City happens without Las Vegas.

Television markets are measured in size, or population. New York is number one, Los Angeles is number two, Chicago number three, and so forth. In early 1985, Lubbock was near market size 120, and Las Vegas was somewhere around 90. In early 2019, Las Vegas is market size 42.

Moving from Lubbock to Las Vegas in the mid-80s meant I was moving up in market size, but not by that much. The perception was that there was a huge difference; Las Vegas was thought of as more of a major sports town. Lubbock is not.

Market size equals revenue. Market size also equals pay, with Las Vegas having a market size barely in the top 100 at the time. I knew I wasn't going to be getting that big of a bump in pay, because it was not that big of a jump in market.

When I accepted the interview, there were certain parameters involved. I flew out for the interview, but I could only visit the station, KVBC, in the morning, because they didn't want the current sports guys to know that they were interviewing replacements. The plan was to fire the two current sports guys and move their current main news anchor over to be sports director. I was being brought in to be the weekend sports anchor, or in other words, the number two guy. That plan gave me more than a hint of what was ahead.

When I accepted the position, I knew I was in for a long stretch of days without a day off. Eventually, I would anchor on weekends, and then be a sports reporter three days during the week, Monday through Friday. The move to transition the main news anchor over to sports director wouldn't happen until after the month of February, which is an important month for ratings. Station management wanted him to remain in the news anchor position because of February ratings.

My first day on the air was Feb. 2, 1985, and I wouldn't have a day off until March. The good thing about working every day was that I would be paid for overtime. I didn't make overtime in Lubbock, because I was strictly salary. I knew I was going to make some good money during that four-week stretch.

KVBC didn't pay a moving company to move me, but they did offer to pay for a rental truck. It was up to me to load my belongings and drive out. The day I was supposed to leave, a major snowstorm hit Lubbock, and stretched all the way past Albuquerque to the west.

It dumped eight inches of snow on Lubbock and most of the state of New Mexico, where the state line is about 90 minutes from Lubbock.

I would have to drive a rented Ryder truck with a trailer connected to the back, on which I had to mount my car. It felt like I was driving an 18-wheeler, which of course, I'd never done. The guy at the Ryder rental place helped secure my car with chains so it wouldn't fall off. I was planning to drive my car from Lubbock to Albuquerque to Phoenix and then up to Las Vegas. The presence of the snow storm meant I couldn't go through the mountains.

I left Thursday morning, planning to get to Las Vegas by noon on Friday. My first day on the air was going to be Saturday at 5 p.m. I was supposed to check into my new apartment on Friday afternoon, and I was going to be on the air, anchoring sports, a little more than 24 hours later. With all that in mind, KVBC would fire the two sports guys after Friday's broadcasts.

Due to the snowstorm, my timetable for travel became much more of a challenge. I had to drive south and detour 12 hours. It took me six hours just to get to Midland/Odessa, a drive that usually took just three hours. I finally arrived in El Paso around midnight, where I found a hotel room. It was too cold to sleep in the car.

I slept for about five hours in El Paso, and then got up before the sun. I traveled to Tucson, and finally got to Phoenix mid-afternoon on Friday. I had rented the apartment in Las Vegas, sight unseen, but it was brand new, so I figured it would be fine. When I got to Phoenix, I called the apartment complex. The office manager at the apartment complex said the office closed at 6 p.m. It's usually a four- to five-hour drive from Phoenix to Las Vegas, so there was no way I was going to make it, even though I didn't know exactly how far it was.

I figured, "You gotta do what you gotta do," so I pressed on. As I got closer to Las Vegas, I saw signs that said, "Hoover Dam, 20 miles," and then "Hoover Dam 10 miles." I'd heard of the Hoover Dam, but I hadn't put two and two together at the time. I didn't realize it was that close to Las Vegas.

I needed to get to Las Vegas, so I kept driving, across the Hoover Dam. I saw total darkness on one side and total darkness on the other side. There were high-beam searchlights coming up from everywhere as I drove across the dam. I was worn out, it was dark out, and I had no idea what was "over the edge" of the Hoover Dam.

About six weeks later, I finally took a daytime trip to the Hoover Dam. I couldn't believe how close I was to the edge. It was good that my drive on that trip was at night, because I would have been freaking out.

When I finally got to Henderson, Nevada, I could see the lights of Las Vegas getting brighter in the distance. I stopped and found a pay phone. It was probably about 7 or 7:30, and I called the television station. I said, "I need to speak with Doug Ballin." He was the news director, the guy who hired me. The producer on the other end said, "Doug called in sick today."

I was thinking, "God, are you sure this is what you want me to do? Did I make the right decision?" The previous 36 hours had been the road trip from hell.

I said, "My name is Al Wallace." She interrupted and said, "Oh, Al Wallace. He told me that you might be calling. He's home. He's got the flu, but here's his home number. Call him." I called Doug at home, and he told me to go to Circus, Circus (one of the casinos there). The station had an account there; I could stay there, and they were expecting me.

I never made it to my apartment that evening, but I checked into the hotel, took a hot bath and had a great meal. I got up the next morning and checked into my apartment. I unpacked and returned the Ryder truck, all by noon. I unpacked a little, and then I went to work to anchor the 5 p.m. and the 11 p.m. sportscasts. That pace went on for 30 days. I never unpacked completely, or really even had a chance to.

On Monday, after my first weekend, just like in most college towns with a college basketball team, head coach Jerry Tarkanian had his weekly press conference for the UNLV Runnin' Rebels. They were "the" sports story and sports team in Las Vegas. The Runnin' Rebels were one of the most popular college basketball teams in the country, just a couple years after stars like Reggie Theus and Sidney Green played there.

While I was in Las Vegas, UNLV quarterback Randall Cunningham was drafted into the NFL by the Philadelphia Eagles. Also while I was in Las Vegas, we hosted an in-studio interview with a 15-year-old tennis prodigy named Andre Agassi.

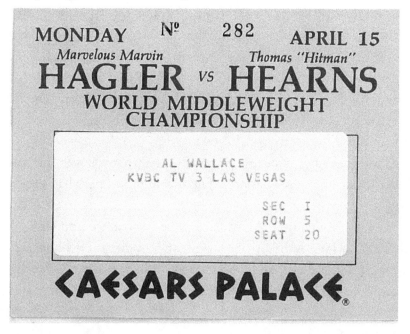

MONDAY   Nº   282   APRIL 15
Marvelous Marvin   *Thomas "Hitman"*
HAGLER *vs* HEARNS
WORLD MIDDLEWEIGHT
CHAMPIONSHIP

AL WALLACE
KVBC TV 3 LAS VEGAS

SEC   I
ROW   5
SEAT   20

‹A‹SARS PALA‹‹.

One of the perks of working in Vegas was covering big-time boxing matches

I knew when I moved to Las Vegas that there would be no Southwest Conference football. There would be no Dallas Cowboys or Houston Oilers. There would be no Texas high school football. The sports climate in Las Vegas was John McEnroe and Jimmy Connors playing a high-stakes tennis match at Caesar's Palace, or maybe a "Marvelous" Marvin Hagler vs. Thomas "Hit Man" Hearns boxing match.

During my three months in Las Vegas, I covered two World Championship boxing matches. During one match, I sat on the first row, right next to the ring. Behind me was movie star and boxing fan Sylvester Stallone. One night I hung out with CNN sports anchor Nick Charles, and I also did a one-on-one interview with boxer Larry Holmes.

That's what my February was like, covering those events and those athletes. I knew that when the college basketball season was over, a large chunk of me being busy would be gone. The summer months, the slow months in a city with no professional sports teams, would be slower. Finding a story here and there in a sports climate I was not familiar with, in a geographical area that I was not familiar with, was going to be more challenging. The bottom line was this: I didn't like Las Vegas. I didn't like living there.

One of the reasons, and one thing I never considered before I accepted the job, was the time difference. Living in Lubbock or Dallas, or now in Kansas City, I was in the Central time zone. That's pretty much like the Eastern time zone, regarding sporting events. There's something to be said about being part of the news-making process.

I could go on the air at 10:20 in Kansas City and the Royals would still be in the top of the eighth with a chance to win, or they would be trying to save the game. One way or another, most often, they would still be "involved" in a game. It was happening while I was on the air, or even preparing for air.

As a sportscaster, you don't get that in the Pacific time zone as often, certainly not in the early months of a year. By the time we did sports on the 11 p.m. newscast, everything had been done for hours. In 1985, there was no Sunday Night Football. NASCAR was nothing like it is now. ESPN SportsCenter and CNN Sports had the only national sports highlights shows.

This was my typical Sunday in the spring of 1985: I'd go to work at 1 p.m., but my mind and my body clock, especially my sports body clock, were telling me it was 3 p.m. Most baseball games were in the seventh inning when I was just showing up at work. Two hours later those games were over. There was no Sunday night baseball. By the time I hit the air at 5:20, most sporting events had been completed. I'd give NBA scores and highlights, but all the games were over.

I'd get done with my sportscast at 5:30, and I wasn't scheduled to hit the air again for almost six hours. I'd spend an hour rewriting and re-racking my sportscast, changing it up a bit, but the facts of the outcome didn't change. At 6:30, I'd go to dinner for an hour. There is no way I could do that in Kansas City, even when we had a big staff. You just didn't have time.

After dinner, I could go to a two-hour movie at 8 p.m., and it was still only 10 p.m. when the movie ended. I'd drive 20 minutes back to work, get back to work by 10:30. I didn't hit the air until 11:20. In some ways the job was challenging, but to me it was very easy and non-challenging.

There wasn't the adrenalin rush that I was used to and desired. It wasn't like a game to me; it was more like two-a-days. It was like practice, and I hated it. I gave serious thought to changing careers, maybe selling insurance or something. I was thinking very seriously about other options after a month of that.

After a couple of weeks, I went to the news director and said, "I'm about to die. I'm exhausted," because I had worked every single day since my arrival. He said, "I understand. Take Tuesday off and we'll get the weekend weather guy to do sports."

I put on my best suit and went to Caesar's Palace. I paid $50 to see Diana Ross. I sat in one of those big booths up front with the high backs. I can tell you that is the last time I drank liquor. Over the last 10 to 15 years, I might have had one or two beers a week, mainly with dinner, but that's the last time I drank hard liquor. I just needed the escape and the getaway.

When I was looking to leave Lubbock, I was looking pretty hard to find another job. I wasn't getting a lot of feedback, but in the late summer and early fall of 1984, I sent resume tapes to TV stations in San Diego, Atlanta and Kansas City. I sent them to all three stations in all three markets. Remember, there was no FOX Network at the time.

I wanted to work in a market that had Major League Baseball, professional football and possibly professional basketball. I wanted major league sports. I also wanted a healthy college climate. And I wanted a station that didn't ignore high school sports, because I was used to the interest in high school sports. I heard back from a couple of stations. including one station in Atlanta. Channel 5 (KCTV) in Kansas City sent me a letter saying, "Don't call us, we'll call you." I didn't hear back from anybody else.

After a month of this pace in Las Vegas, the ratings period ended on Thursday night. I worked Friday, Saturday and Sunday anyway. If I could just survive one more weekend, the news anchor would start on Monday night, which would be my first day off in more than a month.

As I was sitting in the newsroom on Sunday night preparing to do sports, the news anchor called me and told me that he had never observed the setup. He was a news guy, but he didn't know the system or the infrastructure for sports. He said, "I kind of hate to do this, but I'm going to ask you for a favor. Can you come in tomorrow for about an hour and help me get set up? Just help me out for about an hour and kind of show me where a few things are?"

I said, "No problem. I can do that." I could do one extra—One for the Coyotes. It didn't help me at all, but it helped the team. I went in that next day, Monday, and helped him for about an hour.

As I walked out the back door and approached my car, a producer stuck his head out the back door and said, "Hey, Al, you've got a phone call." I went back inside and picked up the phone. The voice on the other end said, "Al, this is Mike Lewis from WDAF-TV in Kansas City. I called your station in Lubbock and the news director there told me that you had moved to this station in Las Vegas. I just want to

63

know if you're still interested in a job here? We'd like to fly you in for an interview."

I had never unpacked all my stuff. I was too busy in the month of February to get to it. I had my waterbed up and that was about it. I was still living out of several suitcases. After I hung up, I walked out that back door and I jumped up and kicked my heels together.

Unfortunately, the earliest WDAF could fly me in for an interview was Tuesday, April 2. Knowing that there *might* be a better opportunity on the near horizon made it much easier to do my job in Las Vegas for another month, especially working just five days a week. I kept thinking, "Just do your job."

One interesting fact that I remember about those three months in Las Vegas was a three-day trip to Yuma, Ariz., to cover the Las Vegas Stars, who were the Triple-A baseball affiliate of the San Diego Padres. The previous fall, the Padres had lost to the Detroit Tigers in the World Series, so the Padres were a pretty big deal, especially in Las Vegas.

A number of players on that Padres team had been minor league players in Vegas, including the late Tony Gwynn and Kevin McReynolds. The Las Vegas audience knew these guys. Recently, I found my press credential from that spring training trip. It was signed by the Padres PR guy, Mike Swanson, who is now the Kansas City Royals VP of Communications.

I went through most of March in 1985 kind of in neutral. I was doing my job, like the trip to Yuma, but I was also hoping for Kansas City. I enjoyed Las Vegas more, hoping that it was temporary. I hung out with coworkers from the television station because they were the only people I knew. They were great friends.

One of those coworkers was our entertainment reporter. He would interview some of the most famous entertainers in the world, who worked on the Las Vegas Strip. We'd ask him, "What are you doing this week?" He'd say, "I've got the Pointer Sisters" or "I've got Paul Anka."

He came to me one day and said, "Sammy Davis Jr. is in town tomorrow night. Do you want to come? You can grip for us, carry the lights or some cables." I jumped at the opportunity.

That next night we went to Sammy Davis Jr.'s nightclub act and stood at the back. We got to see the whole act. I thought, "If my mother could see this." The performance lasted about 90 minutes, and he sang all the favorites: *What Kind of Fool Am I, Candy Man* and *Mr. Bojangles*, just to name a few. After the show, we went backstage so we could do the interview. We went to the dressing room and there were three or four guys—his entourage. One guy took care of his shoes, one has his suit, etc.

Sammy was in the shower, but we went ahead and set up. I don't know if I've ever seen a more confident person in who he was than Sammy Davis Jr. He was so kind and gracious, but more than all that, he was confident. I asked for an autograph, and as requested, he made it out to my mother. I later sent it to her.

I didn't do much talking, because I was clearly star-struck. That night, getting to watch Sammy Davis Jr. perform, and meeting him back stage in his dressing room, was the best night of my stay in Las Vegas. I had an affection for JFK history, and I knew that JFK had a relationship with the "Rat Pack," which included Sammy Davis Jr., Dean Martin, Joey Bishop and Frank Sinatra. To meet a member of the Rat Pack was the neatest part of my stay in Las Vegas.

On April 2, I flew to Kansas City for my interview with WDAF. The plan was to fly in and out on the same day. I got up early to catch a flight, and I got to Kansas City in the mid-morning. Mike Lewis, the news director at WDAF, picked me up at the airport. The first place he took me was to the Truman Sports Complex.

The day before, on April 1, Villanova had beaten Georgetown in the National Championship game of the NCAA Tournament. It was one of the biggest upsets in tournament final history. The Royals were still in training camp in Fort Myers, Florida. At the time, Frank Boal and photographer JW Edwards were covering Spring Training.

When I came into the sports office, I met Gordon Docking. I was sitting there talking with him when the phone rang, and it was Frank. Gordon says, "Yeah, he's here for the interview." They chatted for a moment, and then Gordon said something to the effect of "How about that game last night?" I could hear Frank in the background, "We are national champions! You're never going to take that away from us! I told you!"

Gordon was holding the phone away from his ear. because Frank's a pretty wide-open guy. I thought, "I'm going to be working with this guy if I get the job?" It was all joyous, but that was how I met Frank and Gordon.

Early in the process, Mike and Frank sat down and reviewed about 100 or so resume tapes. Frank looked at them all and he said, "I'll take any one of these three guys." I was one of the three. All three of us came for an interview. The final decision was up to station management and they chose me.

After my visit, Mike called me a week or two later and offered me the job, and I accepted immediately. I think I had a total of six days off before I'd start the new job in Kansas City. I wasn't going to drive and work my first day, and they didn't expect me to. My first day to work in Kansas City was May 8, 1985.

Even though I knew that Las Vegas would be an unknown, I also knew it was a place where I didn't fit. It's Disneyland for grownups. It's a great place to visit, maybe even a great place to live, but it just wasn't for me.

I told myself a couple of things when I moved there. I knew it was the gambling capital of the world, so I told myself I was not going to gamble. The first month I lived there I never did. I never got close to a slot machine or the tables. I hung out with friends, and we'd go into casinos and people-watch. But I never gambled until I realized that Kansas City was a possibility, and even then, I only played the nickel slots.

Friends would tell me if I got an extra $100 and wanted to gamble, fine. They also said, "If you win, don't spend it on a trip, spend it on something tangible. Spend it on a new washing machine, a new dryer, a new oven. Spend it on something that will better your life. Don't blow it."

I never let it get that far. When I was in high school, I worked at a place called Chicken-Go-Go in Mineral Wells. It was a summer job, and I was a fry cook. I told myself that summer, "Don't eat any chicken." When I worked in Las Vegas, I said, "I'm not going to gamble," and I didn't until I found out that Kansas City was a possibility and eventually a reality. The most I ever lost was $5. Gambling just wasn't me.

Las Vegas was a detour I'm glad I took. It's a chapter in my life that made me realize that life is a process that continually requires adjustment. I also learned that sometimes in life being uncomfortable is necessary. You've still got to get up each and every day, pay your dues, live your life, and deal with the consequences of the decisions you've made. If I didn't go into the office on that Monday in early March, when I had already worked a month without a day off, I might never have gotten that phone call from Kansas City.

I wouldn't have gotten that phone call if I hadn't done a little extra, if for just one day, if I didn't do "One for the Coyotes." Through my last day working at WDAF, when I had to go in on a day off, I thought about that day in Las Vegas. Do one more, do a little extra. More often than not, it will pay off.

In the long run, it usually does.

CHAPTER 7

The Border War

WHEN I WAS hired by WDAF in the spring of 1985, the question might have been asked: Why would the news department at WDAF need another sports guy? The answer was they needed another person to do the stories that weren't getting done.

WDAF was the station that aired most Royals games because we had the Royals TV contract. The Royals had been in the playoffs the previous season and in six of the previous nine seasons. When Royals play-by-play man Denny Trease was traveling with the team six months out of the year, there were only two sports guys in the newsroom. They needed another person for local college and high school coverage, and for general assignment sports reporting.

Frank Boal did most of the anchoring. and Gordon Docking did most of the reports from the field. Gordon had a tremendous affection for high school football. When either Frank or Gordon had a day off, there was no one to do just about everything else besides anchoring.

So I was the "sweeper-upper" guy, and I was good with that. In fact, in October 1985, I didn't go to a single Royals postseason game. That was fine with me, because that was not what I was hired to do. I would have loved to have gone, but I was fine.

Bruce Lindsay was working the newsroom assignment desk during the 1985 World Series, and I remember him asking, "You're covering high school football during the World Series?" like it was beneath me. I wasn't just okay with it, I was very okay with it, because I was doing what I was supposed to do. I would have loved to have seen George Brett hit home runs against the Blue Jays, but that's not what I was hired to do.

Following the Royals World Series win in 1985, everyone in our sports department wanted the assignment of covering the Royals during the 1986 Spring Training. Frank Boal, Denny Trease and Gordon Docking all wanted to go to Fort Myers, Florida, and so did I. I'd never been to Royals Spring Training. Yes, the Royals were world champions, but I didn't know what I was missing.

Frank said, "I'm sorry you're not going to be able to go to Spring Training, but if Kansas goes to the Final Four in Dallas, you're going to cover that." We all knew Kansas had a pretty good basketball team that year, with Danny Manning, Calvin Thompson and Greg Dreiling. Kansas indeed qualified for that Final Four, where the Jayhawks lost in the national semifinals to Duke, a team that featured Johnny Dawkins, Danny Ferry and Jay Bilas.

That 1985-86 season was my first taste of Big 8 basketball, and honestly put, I can't remember which arena I visited first: Ahearn Fieldhouse in Manhattan, Kan.; Allen Fieldhouse in Lawrence, Kan.; or The Hearnes Center in Columbia, Mo. I do know I was blown away. I remember a KU vs. K-State game at Ahearn, and doing a live shot about 10 feet from the baseline while the game was going on. There were fans behind the baseline, standing, watching the game. My live shot was right in the middle of those fans during our 10 o'clock sportscast. Everybody was on top of everybody else. Just like the tension in the building, the air was thick, and you couldn't hear.

I remember the crow's nest at Ahearn Fieldhouse where the press box was. It hung from the ceiling. When the crowd was really into the game, the press box shook. I look at Bramlage Coliseum now and still wonder why they didn't just upgrade Ahearn. I, like many others, believe it would have helped preserve the identity of K-State basketball.

For a guy who had been raised on football in the state of Texas—where it's considered a religion all its own—I was overwhelmed by Big 8 basketball. I'd never seen anything like it. I'd never seen college basketball players, in person, with that kind of talent and athleticism.

I didn't realize that these early years of working in Kansas City would become the genesis of my affection for college basketball. In 1985, the Royals were the biggest sports story in town. Nobody wanted the college basketball beat, and I said I would take it. Interestingly, the biggest appeal of the 1986 Final Four for me wasn't that Kansas basketball had qualified; it was the fact that it was in Dallas, which I still considered home.

I remember the Midwest Regional at Kemper Arena, when the clock stopped running with 2:21 left and Michigan State, with guard Scott Skiles, leading KU by four points. The clock stopped running for about 15 seconds, but no time was added to the clock. KU tied the score with nine seconds left, and then won the game in overtime.

Moments like that helped me understand the significance and the impact of Big 8 basketball in Kansas City. The postseason tournament was here, and the three "local" schools were all within a two-hour drive. I ate it up, especially the rivalry between Kansas and Mizzou. My love of history and the relationship between the two states made the rivalry even bigger.

Growing up, my brother Tony and I were basically each other's best friends. He is two years older than I am. As young boys, we had those little plastic Army men. I was the blue Union soldiers and he was the gray Confederate soldiers. I grew up with this uneducated connection to the Civil War. I knew I had the Union soldiers and eventually the Union won the war. Ulysses S. Grant was the head Union general and Robert E Lee was the head Confederate general.

My oldest brother, Carlos, was always quick to point out that even though General Lee lost the war, he was the best-dressed. Ulysses S, Grant was seen as something of a slob. He certainly was not as well-groomed as Robert E Lee.

I loved all those battles that my Union soldiers had won, and Tony loved all the battles that the Confederate soldiers had won. Over time, I detoured to another connection with history and that was American history, the civil rights movement, the history of the 1960s and other significant events.

I've also always had a tremendous appreciation for Texas history. I knew that Texas was rich in history. I knew nothing of Kansas or Missouri history. I remember once, when I was still in high school, a friend talked about some relatives he had near Kansas City. He would come to Kansas City and stay through the summers. He loved the history here.

He would talk about how Lawrence was burned to the ground back in the 1860s. That was because the two states were on opposite sides of the issue concerning slavery.

One of the first things that I noticed when I moved to Kansas City was how different the two states were. When I first moved here, someone told me that because the station itself was in the state of Missouri, it would probably be best if I lived in Missouri. It would be easier at tax time. That's the reason I looked for an apartment in the state of Missouri and that's where I settled, just off the Country Club Plaza near Main Street.

Then I noticed little things like a boulevard called "State Line Road," and that's the true state line, right down the middle of the city. I noticed that on one side was Johnson County, and on the other side was Jackson County.

I also noticed the economic differences. People would tell me that the Kansas City, Missouri school district had just gotten millions of dollars from the federal government to invest in Magnet schools. They didn't have that situation in Johnson County, because those were the better public schools.

I noticed all those things when I first moved here. I recall that in Johnson County, if you wanted to go in a restaurant and buy an alcoholic beverage, you had to be a member of a club. That blew me away. I couldn't go to a restaurant and order a beer with my dinner unless I had a club membership.

It didn't take very long to understand that the differences really manifested themselves easiest in the arena of athletic competition, when the Kansas Jayhawks met the Missouri Tigers. The sport or competition didn't matter. Neither did the location.

Kansas City had a sports rivalry with St. Louis, but meaningful head to head matchups were either rare or non-existent. There were the Royals and the Cardinals, and the Chiefs and the Cardinals, because at the time the football Cardinals were in St. Louis. Those professional teams were all Missouri teams, and they shared common soil. These two universities were from two different states. One state was pro-slavery during the Civil War and one was a free state. It took a while to realize the disdain these two schools had for each other because of their states' histories.

While I was growing up in Texas, we had three state schools that were similar to Mizzou, KU and K-State. We had Texas, Texas A&M and Texas Tech. In my mind, Texas Tech was K-State, Texas A&M was Missouri and the University of Texas was Kansas. They all kind of fit certain social stereotypes. Anyone in Texas will tell you that the Aggies hate the Longhorns, like the Jayhawks hate the Tigers and vice versa. I believe KU and Mizzou hate each other even more.

It was so interesting and enjoyable to watch, because it made the games even more exciting. KU and K-State have their own rivalry. It's a typical in-state rivalry and those exist all over the country. Very few rivalries transcend generations and have so little to do—originally— with athletic events. This rivalry had to do with life-and-death situations. That's where the roots were, back in the mid-1800s, in events that were a big part of leading up to and the Civil War itself.

I fell in love with that history. When they built Arrowhead Stadium and Kauffman Stadium, Jackson County residents got first dibs on tickets. Much of the corporate money is in Johnson County, on the other side of the state line, but that doesn't matter. Jackson County residents—people from Missouri—get first crack at tickets because the stadiums are in Missouri. Modern issues like that currently separate the two states, financially, educationally, socio-economically, and some would say, racially. I found it fascinating. I just fell in love with that mindset.

Here's an example of the sports rivalry, combined with the state rivalry that was manifested in a sports story. Former Missouri head basketball coach Norm Stewart probably didn't have the disdain for the state of Kansas that he portrayed, but when the Tigers played at KU, his team would spend the night in a hotel on the Missouri side of the state line and then drive over to Lawrence the next morning. Stewart didn't do that when he played K-State.

They wouldn't be better prepared to play KU in basketball if they stayed in Missouri than if they stayed in Lawrence, but it was just something about growing up in Sikeston, Missouri. He was a Missourian.

He didn't go out and advertise it, but people knew it. I don't think that Norm actually thought it helped them win or lose, but if he had the option of having it one way, that's the way he was going to have it. He felt it was better to help a business on the Missouri side of the state line, rather than one on the Kansas side of the state line. He loved the fact that when it got reported, it irritated the people in Kansas and pumped up the people in Missouri. He didn't run away from it. He just didn't promote it.

Norm Stewart often referred to the Jayhawks as "Johnny Jayhawks." I heard him say that more than once and he would say it jokingly.

He just fit Missouri so well; I don't think any other basketball coach has since. Being a native Missourian, he represented that school in an almost-perfect way, a hard-hat way, a take-nothing-for-granted, take-no-prisoners, tough mindset.

It was never "just another game" when Norm's Tigers played Kansas. Some coaches may say it, but Norm meant it. Most coaches won't even say it, but Norm did. It was fun to watch Norm coach against Kansas, whether it was against Larry Brown or Roy Williams, right up until the time he retired in 1999.

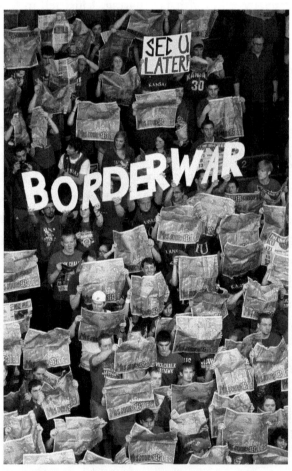

It just meant more when Kansas played Missouri

Football games between Mizzou and Kansas were good, but often not as consequential. I always found the basketball games more heated, and maybe that was because in football, they were in pads and helmets. It was harder to identify with the true heat of the battle.

Basketball is an open-court situation, where you could see and become attached to so much more. You can feel so much more emotion at a basketball game than you do at a football game or another sporting event. You can feel the guys out there in a "non-contact" sport, and you can sense their desire to win. You can see the sweat. You can see how much they care and how badly they want to win and how much they hate to lose, especially to each other.

Midway through the summer of 1994, I was contacted by officials from the Big 8 Conference, to see if I had any interest in hosting a new Big 8 Saturday basketball studio show. Starting in November, I would have to fly to a studio in Charlotte, North Carolina, every Saturday throughout the college basketball season and anchor the show, called "Studio 66," from there.

Station management at WDAF gave me permission to do so, in part because we aired the games and had the Big 8 television contract. I only hosted the studio show for one season, but I continued to work Big 12 basketball games as a sideline and halftime reporter for another five years.

In 1997, I worked the game between Kansas and Missouri, when the Kansas Jayhawks were ranked number 1 in the country and were undefeated when they met the Missouri Tigers in Columbia. Mizzou won the game when Corey Tate hit a shot in overtime. It was during that season that I produced a story on Quantrill's Raid for our WDAF Sunday night sportscast.

I got in touch with a historian named Steve Jansen who was with the Douglas County Historical Society in downtown Lawrence. There's a museum there, and they have some very interesting artifacts from Quantrill's Raid, which took place on August 21, 1863. Among the artifacts was a big bundle of nails from a livery stable, where the heat from the fire set by Quantrill's Raiders was so intense, it melted all the nails together.

I worked the narrations of Steve Jensen into my story, and I also found some old movies that depicted life at that time. I talked to a former Kansas player, Ryan Robertson, who happened to be from St. Charles, Missouri, and I talked with a former Missouri player, Jon Sundvold, who grew up in Blue Springs. Sundvold played for a few years in the NBA and has been a college basketball announcer ever since. I asked both men if the heated history between the two states really played out on the basketball court. Both men said not really. Sundvold specifically said, "Quantrill didn't shoot hoops."

Jensen argued that the rivalry matters more on the Missouri side because the pro-slavery advocates lost the Civil War. It might mean less on the Kansas side because the free state supporters won the war. I believe most fans who follow the recent and present-day rivalry feel more emotional about it than the current players and coaches involved. I find it all fascinating, and that includes the fact that the two schools are no longer members of the same athletic conference.

At the conclusion of the 2011-2012 school year, Missouri left the Big 12 conference and became a member of the Southeastern Conference. The annual athletic matchups between the two schools, that for decades had been commonplace, ceased to exist. No more games, no more matches, none that were regularly scheduled anyway.

The rivalry continues to exist though. So much so that I began to think of it as a "Border War, Cold War." Each school views the other from a distance, looking out of the corner of their eyes. They still compete academically, intellectually and through the improvement and perception of facilities.

Who knows what conference Missouri and Kansas will be aligned with years in the future? They may be aligned again in the same conference. As of right now though, there is *detente*, but I still call it "Border War, Cold War". While working at WDAF, I even had a graphic made up that said, "Border War, Cold War."

My daughter Chase is a graduate of the University of Kansas, and she has never been to Columbia. I've often told her that she's never going to find two towns more different than Columbia and Lawrence. Each town has its own persona and mindset. Even with the separation of affiliation that came with conference realignment in 2012, I still find the rivalry fascinating.

As a reporter and journalist, I always preferred a story that transcended the arena of competition. My friend Bill Jones is working in Dallas, and when he found out that Barry Switzer got the head coaching job with the Dallas Cowboys, he said, "This is great, this guy is going to say something different every day. We're going to have news every day about something interesting that he's said. This is great."

No reporter wants a boring coach, or boring subject matter. As a sports anchor and reporter, I always wanted something or someone interesting to report on. The more interesting and diverse the subject matter, the better the story.

A great example of that was the Border War football matchup in 2007. There were many benign games between Kansas and Missouri over the years when both were in the Big 8, That 2007 game and the hype surrounding it was unbelievable. It was dubbed the "Armageddon Game," because Kansas was ranked No. 2 in the country, and Missouri was ranked No. 1 and they were playing for first place in the Big 12 North.

It was never difficult for me, as a sports journalist, to separate my "fandom" of Kansas basketball from my on-air presentation. For a number of years, I watched Anthony Peeler play high school basketball in Kansas City. I was a huge Anthony Peeler fan. Peeler played in an era of Missouri basketball that featured names like Mike Sandbothe, Greg Church, and Derrick Chievous.

I loved covering those teams. I liked those Missouri teams because they were tough. I think more often than not, they got the better of Kansas because of their toughness. Kansas could win a game against Missouri, but I rarely thought the wins were spectacular. A win almost always seemed to mean more to Missouri.

The video files in our sports department at WDAF for Kansas were twice as big as they were for K-State or Mizzou for two reasons: geography and the success of Kansas basketball. It was noticeably more significant to our viewing audience. Some viewers would just as soon see a Kansas loss as a victory by their own team.

We put those things on videotape and the tapes would have a number. The KU file was up to 86. Mizzou was at 47 and K-State was at 44. Almost twice as much Kansas video existed because of the history and the news concerning the importance of Kansas basketball and the geography.

A particular part of the history of college basketball is unique to the area of eastern Kansas and western Missouri, and the college basketball town that Kansas City has become. Local basketball fans are blessed to have three major universities in the region. For an extended period of time, each school, Kansas, Kansas State and Missouri, hosted two basketball games each season that involved the other two.

Very few would argue that a contest between Kansas State and Missouri carried the same intensity that a contest with Kansas did or does. For me, the interest in Kansas basketball has overshadowed any other sport that I ever covered as a sports journalist.

CHAPTER 8

Kansas Basketball

I AM A fan and follower of everything connected to Kansas basketball. I graduated from Texas Tech, and I still root for the Red Raiders. I'm thrilled that they reached their first Final Four in 2019. As a fan, I can enjoy that without having to think about how I'd report it.

But I've spent most of the last 34 years in Kansas City, and my fondness for Kansas basketball has blossomed over the years.

There are a lot of reasons for that statement, and most of them have to do with family, friends and history. All the local schools have history, but it's hard to argue that the history of Kansas basketball isn't the most enriching.

Before I moved to Kansas City, I never realized that James Naismith, the man who invented the game of basketball, had coached at Kansas. I never knew that Phog Allen, the father of college basketball coaching, had coached at Kansas. I had heard of both Adolph Rupp and Dean Smith, but never knew they had both played at Kansas. Once I started adding it all up, I was drawn to Kansas. If Missouri or Kansas State had had that history. I would have had the same affection there.

Missouri has never been to the Final Four. Kansas State has been four times, but none since 1964. Kansas State has been tantalizingly close, reaching the Elite 8 and falling to an underdog in the NCAA Tournament in both 2010 and 2018. While K-State fell short in 2018, Kansas reached the Final Four, qualifying for a 15th time.

My love of history, and this sport that means so much to this area, drew me in. Kansas City, to me, is a college basketball town. Evidence is the rivalries that exist among these three schools, and the way it captures the attention of the entire area.

Kansas is different when it plays K-State. Missouri was different when its teams played K-State. Kansas was different when it played Missouri. They all shared a rich, regional college basketball history. Over time, in my opinion, the connection was distinct from other sports dynamic in the region.

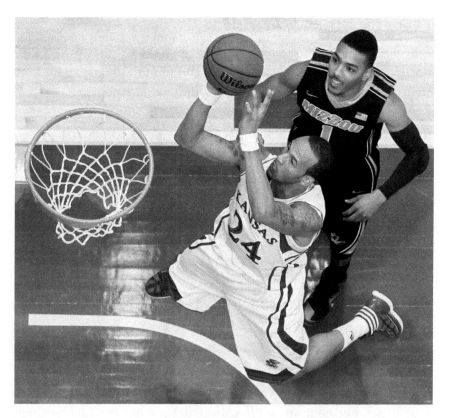

The action was fierce when KU and Mizzou played on the hardwood

Growing up in Texas, I never imagined the significance of another sport other than football. In Texas, no sport could compare, importance-wise, to football. When I moved to Kansas City and realized how much college basketball was in the fabric of the states of Kansas and Missouri, and the three major universities in the region, I was amazed.

It took time to educate myself, and to process the effects of several seasons of competition between the schools involved. It was something I had to experience. It took more than watching one game or one full season from press row. Sure, a game's fun, where one team has to win and one team has to lose. A rivalry, however, is manufactured through time. Winning, losing and perspective help define the intensity of the rivalry.

Big 8 basketball was something different from anything I had experienced prior to 1985. Each school had a separate identity, highlighted by the coaches and high-profile players on the rosters. I remember K-State's Mitch Richmond scoring 36 points at Allen Fieldhouse in 1988. KU had won in Manhattan, and the Wildcats came to Lawrence and returned the favor.

Kansas, ultimately, might have been the best team in the country in 1988, but throughout that season they weren't the best team *in the state of Kansas*. Among the three schools—Kansas, Missouri and K-State—KU was given the longest odds of having success in the 1988 NCAA Tournament. Missouri had a pretty good team, and K-State had a pretty good team that had beaten Kansas twice that year.

I got the assignment of covering Kansas during the first stop of the NCAA Tournament in Lincoln, Nebraska. In that regional, Pittsburgh was a No. 2 seed, North Carolina State was a No. 3 seed, while Kansas was the No. 6 seed.

It is a three-hour drive between Kansas City and Lincoln, and I was traveling with photographer Scott DeJong. On the way, we hit a huge snowstorm. We stopped and checked into a hotel, because we couldn't go any farther. We got up the next morning and finished the trip.

Kansas was banged up, barely given a chance to advance to the Sweet 16. In the first game the Jayhawks beat 11-seed Xavier, while North Carolina State lost its first game in an upset to 14-seed Murray State. So KU got to play Murray State instead of North Carolina State in the second round. Kevin Pritchard, the KU point guard had an injured knee, and he survived that first game and gave a shot of adrenaline to the entire team.

With the two wins, KU advanced to the Sweet 16 in Pontiac, Michigan. Purdue was the heavy favorite to win two games there as the top-seeded team in the whole tournament. KU beat Vanderbilt and future NBA player Will Perdue, when Danny Manning just did everything. He made Perdue look silly. In the second game, K-State upset Purdue, setting up the fourth Sunflower Showdown of the season (they also met in the Big 8 tournament).

K-State and KU would play for the right to advance to the Final Four in Kansas City, and were set to play on a Sunday. On the afternoon before, we took our satellite truck to the K-State hotel. Head coach Lon Kruger had agreed to do a live shot with me at 5 o'clock. Coach Kruger came down to the hotel lobby, which was packed with K-State fans. He was so forthcoming during the live interview. All the K-State fans were nice and gracious, not raucous. They were quiet enough to let us do a two- or three-minute interview live back to Kansas City.

That set the stage for the regional championship game on Sunday. I had figured KU's luck had run out, because they had gotten so many breaks along the way during the tournament. Some people thought they might not even make the tournament, but they got a pretty high seed, relatively speaking.

K-State was the first opponent that KU played in that tournament that had a better seed. That NC State upset really helped KU, because the Wolfpack, coached by Jim Valvano, had a really good team.

Even then, some will say that K-State spent all their bullets in the late Friday night victory over Purdue. As it turned out, Kansas won the regional championship game over K-State, behind a great performance by little-known reserve Scooter Barry. He was best known as the son of NBA legend Rick Barry. Danny Manning also had another great game.

After the game, we first tried to get into the Kansas locker room, but it was packed. I told my photographer, "We can come back; we've got to cover both teams." So, we made our way into the K-State locker room. It was like a morgue in there. We were the only Kansas City TV crew in there for at least five minutes. I remember talking to Lon Kruger and a couple of players who were just devastated.

I realized that any postgame report that I did had to be a 50-50 story. KU's season was going to continue, but K-State's season had ended. How unfortunate that it had to end the way it did, to their cross-state rival.

At this point in my career, I knew this rivalry was different from KU vs. Mizzou, but to me it was just as rich. I had some friends who were K-State grads. and I could only imagine how they were feeling, because that Elite 8 game will forever say that Kansas beat K-State.

Kansas made it to the Final Four, where they got a rematch with Duke, who beat them in the 1986 Final Four. The Jayhawks won the 1988 national semifinal game, then won an epic battle against Oklahoma for the national championship.

That was about as enjoyable a week as I've ever had in covering sports, because that national championship game wasn't the only major sporting event in Kansas City that day. Prior to tipoff, the Royals opened the season at Kauffman Stadium against the Toronto Blue Jays. George Bell hit three home runs and the Blue Jays won.

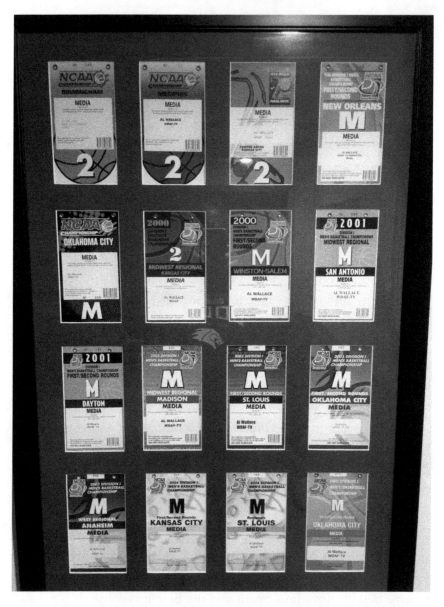

Al rarely missed a KU game in the NCAA Tournament

Looking back to when I applied to work at WDAF, the reason I chose Kansas City was I wanted to cover professional sports and I wanted a college atmosphere. That weekend, I was like, "Man, you have died and gone to heaven." That day of the championship game summed it up. The 50th Final Four and all that went with it, a local team winning it, and the start of the Major League Baseball season. It was fantastic. To have Kansas win, just cemented that Kansas basketball was truly something special, something unique.

While that day, and that week, will stay in my memory forever, it didn't take long for Kansas basketball coach Larry Brown to say, "I'm leaving," followed by "Wait, no I'm not," then, "Oh yeah, I am." He originally accepted the job to return to UCLA, where he coached from 1989-91. The UCLA athletic department had the press conference scheduled and announced when Brown called to tell them he had changed his mind.

Before Kansas fans could get comfortable in the knowledge that their coach was sticking around, Brown announced that he was, in fact, leaving, this time to take the head coaching job for the San Antonio Spurs in the NBA.

That was the first time I experienced one of the things I really don't like about covering television sports. It's best not to get emotionally attached to a player or a coach, because most often they will treat it like a business. I guess they have to do what's best for them and their family.

I tell my daughter Chase, "Don't fall in love with the team or the coach, fall in love with the school, and what that team represents for the school." The players want to be in school a year or two and they're gone. The coaches are dedicated to coaching at that school, until they're not. The emotional attachment, those first couple of weeks after the Final Four in 1988, was my first real taste of the fact these are just people. They're not gods. They're tremendous athletes and coaches, but they're also just people.

There were a couple of years of hiatus from Kansas basketball for me. Kansas was on probation for the NCAA tournament in 1989, and

I followed Missouri in the tournament that season. Norm Stewart had been diagnosed with cancer and Rich Dailey had taken over the coaching reins. Anthony Peeler as a freshman on that Missouri team. I followed them to Dallas and then to Minneapolis where they lost to Syracuse and Derrick Coleman.

The next year, I moved to Dallas and missed Kansas basketball to a very large extent. I had grown an affection there. I saw only one Kansas game that year, and that was when the Jayhawks played SMU in Moody Coliseum.

I missed Kansas playing in the tournament in 1990 when they lost to UCLA, and that's the last road game, outside of the Kansas City area, that I missed with Kansas in the NCAA tournament, until March of 2018.

As much as my love of history drove my relationship to Kansas basketball, my relationship with each of the coaches—Larry Brown, Roy Williams and Bill Self—has deepened it tremendously.

I wouldn't say it was a working relationship with Brown. He recognized me and I recognized him. If Kansas had a 7 or 7:30 p.m. tip at the Fieldhouse, he would do live shots with Frank Boal at 6 o'clock, about an hour before the game. Brown's time was valuable, and he was taking time to be with us. Frank would have to be hooked up and ready to go live.

We didn't want Coach Brown to be sitting there for 10 minutes, so I was the runner to get him. I'd get Coach Brown at the locker room door, with help from sports information, and I'd run him out to Frank. He'd do the minute and a half interview, but he'd only be gone from the locker room for three minutes. I'd also gotten to know assistant coaches Alvin Gentry and R.C. Buford a little bit too.

Coach Brown was always accessible. As time went on, as we got closer to 1988, that kind of access went away. Then, obviously, he went away. There was, however, a connection that our station had cultivated covering Kansas basketball. In qualifying for the 1986 Final Four,

Kansas had already reconnected with its championship tradition.

I worked in Dallas from July 1989 until August 1990, a total of 13 months. While there, the Spurs came to town and played the Mavericks. Prior to the game they had a shoot-around, and I was just sitting there on the sideline. Larry Brown saw me. He just walked over and said, "How're you doing?" He shook my hand because he recognized me.

With Brown, it was more of a friend thing than a working relationship, because the media at that time was so different. That's about as close as I got with Larry Brown. Frank was the connection, so much more than I was.

With head coaches Larry Brown and Roy Williams, Kansas basketball regained its balance on the national stage. There was still a lot more attention from our sports department on the Royals and the Chiefs. When I got back to Kansas City in late 1990, I had a strong desire to reconnect with Kansas basketball. As far as I was concerned, that assignment was still open.

So in 1991, I traveled with Kansas to Louisville, Kentucky, where they played New Orleans, and then Pitt during the first weekend of the NCAA Tournament. KU was the No. 3-seed, but I remember telling a senior by the name of Mike Maddox, on the players' day off in between games, "I don't think you guys can beat Pitt."

He was like "Really?" To this day, whenever I see him, that conversation inevitably comes up. I remember seeing him during the 2014 World Series at Kauffman Stadium. Mike brought his family over to the stadium and we talked about it a little bit, the fact that I didn't think KU could beat Pitt back in 1991. Boy, was I wrong.

From Louisville, they went to Charlotte, North Carolina, to qualify for the Final Four. In the first game they beat No. 2 seed Indiana and Bobby Knight. In the Elite 8, they beat No. 1 seed Arkansas, coached by Nolan Richardson. The Jayhawks were underdogs in both games and wound up winning.

One of the most memorable moments about that trip was the fact that the regional was in Charlotte. Roy Williams' mom was at the team hotel and I interviewed her. Shortly after the interview, Roy came down from his room and hugged her in the hotel lobby. Just a few years after that she passed away and everybody realized how close they were. I knew that Roy grew up in Asheville, North Carolina, which is where my father was born and raised. I hadn't told that to Roy at the time, but I told that to his mom.

A week later in the national semifinal game, Kansas beat Roy's alma mater, North Carolina, coached by his mentor, Dean Smith. Then, on a Monday night in Indianapolis, Kansas lost to Duke in the national championship game.

My most memorable part of that was after the loss to Duke, I was standing with a gaggle of reporters behind one of those big blue curtains. Those curtains quickly parted at one point and rushing through came a squadron of Secret Service agents. Right in the middle of them walked Dan Quayle, the Vice President of the United States, a former senator from Indiana.

He walked five feet from me, surrounded by all those secret service guys. One agent's coat flew open and I could see a machine gun. We were all in such shock because it was all happening so quickly. Still, I thought, "Why not?" So I shouted, "What did you think of the game?" Dan Quayle, the Vice President of the United States, looked straight at me, and with his thumb up, he said "Great game!" We had that on camera and that led our newscast the next day.

After the game, Roy Williams started getting emotional. He talked about how good a season it was, and he cried. All those things helped tie me to Kansas basketball. I saw all of it as history. North Carolina, Duke, Charlotte, Roy's mom, all those things drew me in.

I will say that I put Roy Williams on a pedestal, because he won so many games, and was the caretaker of such a valuable part of the sports culture around the Kansas City TV market. Roy had a lot of focus on his team and his program, and he was a great coach.

Roy's love for his kids, and the emotion he showed, was very real. Some people thought it was staged, but he really loved the kids who played for him. Sometimes you can say you love them too much.

Roy always held a press conference after the game. About 90 percent of the time, he would allow me to meet with him in the hallway for a quick one-on-one interview. We did that for years.

Roy asked me once to come over and talk to the basketball team about how to relate to the media. It was Blair Kerkhoff and me. We were guest speakers at Hadl Auditorium, speaking to a freshman class that included Ryan Robertson and Paul Pierce. We talked with them about how to conduct an interview and how to see things from our side.

Roy wanted his players to understand why we asked the questions we did, and why we thought they were relevant. Roy was the one who got that going. He was a great basketball coach. Who would have ever thought that when he left things would get better for Kansas? There was so much anxiety when he considered the North Carolina job in 1999. Then, when he accepted the job in 2003, the college basketball world seemed to end for Kansas fans...for about four days. Then, in stepped Bill Self.

Self was a grad assistant at KU my first year in Kansas City in 1985. I don't think I ever met him as I barely knew my way around. I recognized Self later as an assistant coach at Oklahoma State. I didn't notice him much until he took his Tulsa team in 2000 to the Elite 8 and lost to North Carolina.

After that, Self took over the program at Illinois. In the spring of 2001, Kansas played Illinois in the NCAA Tournament in San Antonio. Self's team throttled KU. They were more physical, they defended and they out-rebounded Kansas. They were just better.

In 2002, the two teams meet in Madison, Wisconsin, in the Sweet 16. The day before they met. I was in the Illinois locker room. Self was chatting with a bunch of reporters, kind of off-the-cuff. I walked by the huddle and he said, "Hey, man!" He broke up whatever he was talking about with the reporters, and came up to me and very enthusiastically said, "How're you doing?" You'd think he had known me forever.

When he was up for the Kansas job after Roy Williams left, I started thinking, "I hope they get this guy." On April 21, 2003, Bill Self was introduced as the eighth head coach in Kansas basketball history. He agreed to be a guest at the top of our 6 o'clock newscast. KU basketball SID Mitch Germann was going to bring him to our live location.

I was sitting there at the top of the newscast doing headlines, and the producer told me in my ear, "You'll be on in five seconds."

I could see Self down at the end of the court. I said, "Mitch, hurry up," but that wound up on the air. I recovered quickly and said, "If you'll stick with us for 30 seconds, you'll meet the new basketball coach at KU." That turned out to be the perfect tease, because Self heard me say that and he rushed over. He sat down and did a live interview with me.

The great thing about our relationship is when I talk with Self, we rarely talk much basketball. After he lost that first round game to Bucknell in 2005 to end his second season, I wrote him a note that just said, "Hang in there. You'll get over this." He didn't write me back.

I know that year was really tough for him. Not only did his team lose in the first round in a major upset, the school he left, Illinois, faced the school coached by his KU predecessor, North Carolina, for the national championship.

Self had a mid-summer press conference, so I went over to Lawrence for that. Afterwards we started talking. He told me that Billy Gillispie, his former assistant at Illinois, grew up in a small town very near Mineral Wells. He said, "Billy Clyde is from Graford, Texas."

I don't know how Self knew I was from Mineral Wells. I started talking about growing up and then I said something about Possum Kingdom Lake, which is in north-central Texas. Self said, "You went to PK?" No one knows to call it PK unless you've been there. He didn't call it Possum Kingdom Lake, he said "PK."

I said, "Are you kidding me? You've been to PK." He said, "Man, I'm from Oklahoma City. We used to go there all the time and go cliff diving."

So, a lot of our relationship has not been about basketball. It's been about the people that we are. Bill Self such a people-person.

I know of at least three or four different occasions during a tournament where Kansas played a game and the only opportunity for the team to visit with their relatives was when they were getting on the bus. WDAF photographer JW Edwards would usually shoot video and we would always watch Self interact with the families. He knows every family member's name. It's like he never forgets a name, or a person, or an event.

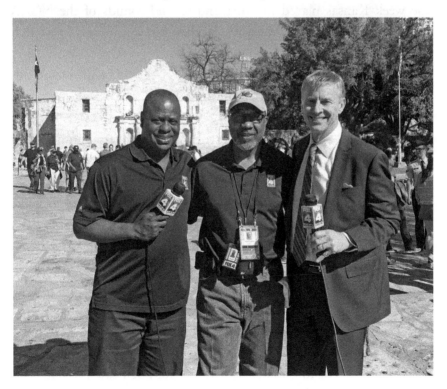

Covering the Jayhawks allowed Al to travel to some
great destinations like San Antonio

There are a few great personal examples that stick out in my mind too. I want to say the first was KU's 2009 preseason media day. JW Edwards had been out for two or three months because he had been treated for prostate cancer. I was standing there outside the media room, and Self walked into Allen Fieldhouse. He immediately said, "Hey Man, what's up?" I said, "Coach, you may not know this, but this is JW's first day back because he's been treated for cancer."

When JW walked up, Coach Self said, "This can wait." He gave us a 20-minute tour of the brand new facilities, including the locker room and the office. We didn't take the camera. He wanted to do that for JW, just to say, "Welcome back."

The most personal example happened in the spring of 2018. It was the week Kansas played the first and second rounds of the NCAA tournament in Wichita. My sister, Jacelyn, had a routine surgery that went bad.

I told JW before we traveled down there, "I may be distracted this week because my sister is in bad shape." Twice, away from the court, Bill Self said to JW, "Hey, JW, how're you doing? Where's your buddy?" JW would say, "He's back at the hotel," and the conversation never got past that. JW knew that I was struggling and didn't want to be at the arena any more than I had to.

While we were in Wichita my sister passed away. I had to make the decision—and it was a no-brainer—to not go to the next NCAA site with KU, which was Omaha for the Sweet 16. That was the first NCAA tournament game away from Kansas City for Kansas basketball that I did not sit courtside since 1990. There were three games I didn't see Kansas play in the tournament, but they were all games played in Kansas City. I thought someone else from the station deserved a chance to go.

When JW got to Omaha with John Holt, Self saw JW and said, "Where's your guy?" I was at home packing to leave for Dallas early the next morning to go to my sister's funeral. JW said, "Coach, he's not going to be here, he had a death in the family." Self said, "What happened?" So JW told him.

At midnight that night, I got a text from Self. He said, "I'm really sorry for your loss. I know how much these games mean to you. We'll do our best to win." I texted him back. I said, "Coach, you don't know how much this means."

I told him a little bit about my sister who was a single mom with three kids. The two girls went to Baylor on math scholarships, and my nephew went to Texas A&M. I also said, "FOE," which means "Family Over Everything." He knew what that meant. Not even Kansas basketball was as important as my sister.

I guess my absence was noticeable in Omaha, because when I arrived at the Final Four in San Antonio, I had numerous reporters and photographers offer me their condolences. It made me feel really good and appreciated.

The final example was my last game at Allen Fieldhouse working for WDAF in December 2018, when KU hosted Villanova. The only person who knew that fact and had an opportunity to tell Self was Chris Theisen, the sports information director. KU won the game. Self just usually hangs out with reporters a little bit after the press conference and then goes back in the locker room. But following that press conference, he walked straight over to me and said, "Big Al." I knew that he knew.

I said, "Coach, do you need anybody to wash towels or anything?" He said, "You're always welcome over here." We didn't have to talk about nuts and bolts or anything.

JW was standing there and he said, "Al wouldn't want me to do this, but Coach, can I get a picture?" Self said, "Absolutely." He knew that was my last game. We've texted a little bit since then. I texted him after KU beat Tech. I said, "You beat my alma mater." He said, "You need to get over here." He's a class act.

Several years ago, I was emceeing a dinner where he was the guest speaker. I asked him in private, "How do you do it?" He said, "What are you talking about?" I said, "You've got these 18-, 19- or 20-year-old kids and you never know what they're doing. You've got 12 or 13 guys. You have to look after them. You never know what they're doing. The phone rings in the middle of the night, how do you do it? I know you make big money, but how do you do it?"

He said, "I love it. You can make a difference in people's lives, in a player's life. You can help them, and you can help their families all through basketball. I love it."

College basketball. I love it too.

CHAPTER 9

The Fieldhouse

IT WASN'T OFTEN over the years that Frank Boal would tell me, "Here's a story I want you to do." Usually—95 percent of the time—he would allow me to find my own stories. Once, during my early years at WDAF, he read about a sportswriter who was working his way across the country writing stories about college basketball. That writer was going to be at Allen Fieldhouse covering a Kansas basketball game.

During the interview, he said something to the effect of, "Where else in America can you get to a college basketball game and drive up Naismith Drive?" That kind of hit home. I knew who James Naismith was, but that question really connected with me as to the importance of Naismith and his relationship to Lawrence, Kansas.

At the time there was no ESPN College Gameday or anything like that. A lot of what you learned about the game of college basketball, you had to find out on your own. I started digging a little bit. Through time and through osmosis, I realized just how significant the arena called Allen Fieldhouse was. There were so many ties to the history of the game itself.

One of the historical connections was Max Falkenstein, who broadcasted Kansas sporting events for 60 years. Max went to elementary school with my late mother-in-law, Marie Brohammer. Back in the late 1940s, right after he returned from serving in the Army Air Corps, Max was working at WREN radio. He gave a young guy from Alma, Kansas, by the name of Jack Dale some broadcasting tips.

Jack became the play-by-play guy for the Texas Tech Red Raiders from 1953 to 2003. He broadcast Texas Tech football and basketball games, more than a half century before Kansas grad Brian Hanni broadcast Texas Tech basketball games.

I was at the Fieldhouse in 2002, and Texas Tech was in Lawrence to play Kansas. I was talking with Jack when Max walked over. They both pointed at me and say, "You know this guy?" We all burst out laughing. Then they told me the story of their friendship that started back in the late 1940s. Then I remembered that Jack was from a small town in Kansas. He said, "Max helped me start my career." Jack has passed away since, but he was great as the voice of Texas Tech football and basketball for decades.

Things like that put into perspective how important people are, as well as the connections and relationships they develop throughout life. The games come and go. The players and coaches come and go, but they all leave a mark. They all have a legacy. They all leave their impression: points scored, games won or relationships developed. It all comes back to the people being people. Those two guys, veteran broadcasters, just exuded respect for each other. It was a brief two-minute conversation and they both went on that day to do their respective jobs. They had games to broadcast.

Another part of my appreciation was simply the games themselves, and how important these athletic events are to the people who follow them. This isn't exclusive to Kansas basketball. One of the things that separates different sports is the frequency of games. There is only one football game a week, so each one seems more precious. Teams play baseball almost every day. You can lose two or three in a row, but you can also win two or three in a row and it can all happen within the span of one week.

Basketball, of all the sports, is where you can be the most connected to the action. There's not the barrier of distance you have with baseball and football. There's not the barrier of camouflage of a uniform and a helmet that you have with football. This is especially true at Allen Fieldhouse, where you can attend a game and feel like you're part of the game because you're right on top of the action.

It's been that way for more than 40 years because of upgrades and renovations to the original structure. Allen Fieldhouse, which first hosted a college basketball game in 1955, still has the charm it had more than six decades ago.

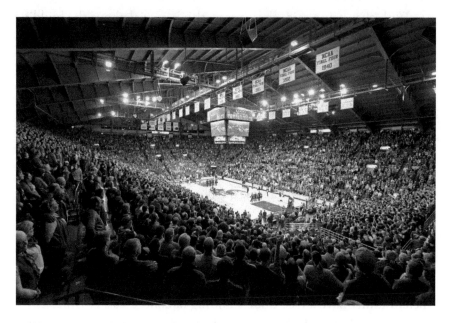

There's no atmosphere in college basketball like Allen Fieldhouse on gameday

When you attend a game at Allen Fieldhouse as a fan, you often feel like you're part of the game itself. It can be so loud and yet intimate. That's what makes it a special place, along with its history and its connection to the man who invented the game.

It's interesting that the only coach in Kansas history to have a losing record was Dr. Naismith himself. It's a quirky fact and really a subject for a different book.

Each school's history, every little nugget of history, separates it from all others. I respect them all. No one school or one team owns college basketball. You can't judge it that way. I tell my kids, "Just because something is not important to you, doesn't mean it is not important to someone else."

My daughter Chase will say, "I hate that player," and "I don't like the way he plays." I'll tell her, "The guy just scored 18 points. You've got to give him that."

With that being said, there's something special about the building itself—Allen Fieldhouse. All arenas are different empty from what they are when they're full. When Ahearn Fieldhouse in Manhattan was empty, well, they called it "the barn" for good reason. On game day, when the K-State Wildcats were playing well, it was amazing.

But when you walk into an empty Allen Fieldhouse, it's almost as if you hear the echoes of the fans, doing the Rock Chalk Chant. You look up and see the sign that says, "Pay Heed To All Who Enter, Beware of the Phog." The walls, the aisles, the bleachers, the seats, they all speak to you.

There's something about an empty Allen Fieldhouse that is intimidating. Then you put 16,300 fans in there and it's even more so. I didn't sense it initially, but over time I did, because when I first got there, I didn't have a true understanding of college basketball.

I knew Lubbock Municipal Auditorium—"the Bubble"—that seated 8,400. I knew that KU and K-State had a rivalry. I decided to watch it, absorb it, process it and try to understand it. The connection between the two schools and the two fieldhouses really ended in 1988 when Bramlage Coliseum was under construction and then became functional in 1989.

I have a good friend whose brother is an architect and was part of the construction team that built Bramlage Coliseum. Back in 1988, both brothers were in Manhattan for different business reasons when Bramlage was under construction. The older brother, the architect, said to his younger brother, "Come on over and I'll show you the new K-State arena."

They were there in the late afternoon or early evening, and they wound up being the only two people in the yet-to-be completed building. They're both Kansas grads, and they decided to go down to the floor of the arena and do the "Rock Chalk Chant."

To this day, they believe that's why it took decades for K-State to beat Kansas at Bramlage Coliseum. That's what makes a rivalry: to think, and in some ways to believe, that something like putting a curse on an arena is possible.

Fortunately—I believe—Kansas has never opted to build a new arena. Instead, resources have been committed to keep Allen Fieldhouse modern, yet historic.

That's what makes the game-day atmosphere at Allen Fieldhouse so great. It all starts with anticipation. When you first walk in, you feel as if you're about to witness something special. It doesn't matter if it's an exhibition game against Fort Hays State or a non-conference game against Louisiana-Lafayette or if K-State is coming to town. The anticipation is real.

I've never seen fans at a venue so busy away from the court before tip-off. Most of the pregame activity can be tied to fans being able to appreciate and absorb so much of the history of KU sports. The Booth Family Hall of Athletics was built not just to connect you to the event, but to the school and its athletic past.

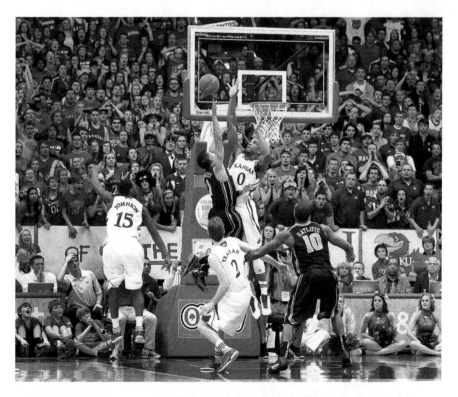

KU's defense stepped up in the last game vs. Mizzou at the Fieldhouse

The 2019 game day presentation obviously is different than it was in 1985. I've told athletic officials at Kansas on numerous occasions, "I don't know who is doing your pre-game or in-game video, but they deserve a raise every year." The game day presentation connects the past to the present, through sight, sound and the live event itself. It connects the student body, the old fan, the young fan and the new fan. It's all geared toward being an antagonist against the opposing team. The crowd at Allen Fieldhouse is the ultimate sixth man of college basketball.

It's an atmosphere that's unique to all of college basketball. Over the years, you may have heard people say, "Maybe we need a new place." The talk never lasts long. WDAF sports reporter Jason Lamb once produced a story that included the original blueprints of Allen Fieldhouse. It's an arena that has withstood the test of time. It's not just the home for Kansas basketball, it's become a destination, even a "bucket list" place.

I was at the Fieldhouse for a game once in the mid-90s, when Roy Williams had golfer Fred Couples as a special guest. Couples was also good friends with baseball hall of famer George Brett, who occasionally would come to basketball games. Couples had to make it to Allen Fieldhouse. I recall thinking, "What is Fred Couples doing at the Fieldhouse? Tom Watson, sure, but Fred Couples?"

When you go to the Fieldhouse now, you can see Hollywood stars like Rob Riggle and Jason Sudeikis. If you went into Bill Self's office, you'd see autographed pictures of Self with President Obama or Bruce Springsteen. Just like a famous athlete who transcends his sport and connects beyond that sport to the culture of the time, Bill Self is more than a just college basketball coach.

That's another thing that makes Bill Self unique. He transcends his job description. He has reached so many other parts of society and culture that people find important, significant or entertaining. That is truly special. Self is quick to point out that it's not him, or even Kansas basketball. It's Allen Fieldhouse itself, and the experience of going to see a college basketball game there.

I realized over time that while anchoring sports from the studio, I would refer to Allen Fieldhouse simply as, "The Fieldhouse." I had stopped calling it "Allen Fieldhouse." I realized that maybe 10 years ago. It had become second nature. I trusted that our audience knew what I was talking about and I just kind of left it there.

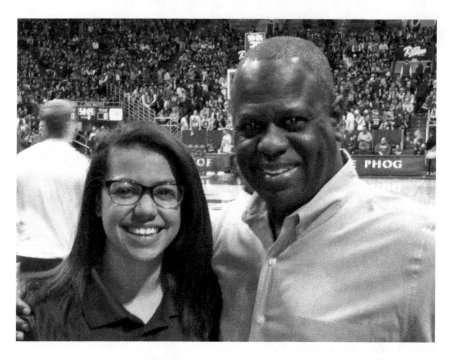

Having Chase in the KU pep band made gameday even more enjoyable

For a four-year stretch of covering games at the Fieldhouse, from the fall of 2013 to the spring of 2017, my daughter Chase was part of the Kansas basketball pep band. Growing up, Chase resented KU basketball. My wife, Marlena, was born in Lawrence and raised on a farm south of Lawrence. She insisted that both of our daughters be born in Lawrence, though we lived in Prairie Village and Overland Park, Kansas, respectively, when they were born. I had to drive my wife—in labor—to Lawrence so our daughters would be born there.

In 2003, the last season that Roy Williams coached at Kansas, Chase was 7-years old. KU played in the Big 12 tournament in Dallas, and I was gone for six days. The next week, Kansas played in the first and second rounds of the NCAA tournament in Oklahoma City, and I was gone five or six more days. I came back and got a suitcase full of clean clothes and followed Kansas to Anaheim, where they beat Duke and Arizona to qualify for the Final Four.

When Kansas beat Arizona to win the West Regional, Marlena found Chase kicking and screaming on the floor when the final buzzer went off on television. She knew I was going to be gone for another week. She wanted Kansas to lose, just so I'd stay home. I was gone basically an entire month. Chase didn't mind Kansas basketball, but she hated the month of March because I was always gone.

Over time, Chase became a talented clarinet player. She loved going to band camp at Kansas, so during her junior year of high school she decided that she wanted to study music at the University of Kansas. That was the only reason she wanted to enroll at KU.

She knew everyone and every nook and cranny at Murphy Hall, which is the School of Music at Kansas. During the summers she practically lived there. She had to audition to be accepted into that school of music, and she passed that with flying colors.

During her high school years, there were numerous occasions when she would have to be at a music festival or event at KU. If there was inclement weather, I'd drive her over the night before. We'd stay at the downtown Marriott in Lawrence so she'd stand a better chance of being on time the next day.

When she made the decision to attend Kansas, I told her, "If you're going to go to KU and study music, it would be best for your social life if you learned something about Kansas basketball. Otherwise, you're going to be ostracized."

I still had to talk her into trying out for pep band. In high school, Chase was a four-time all-state clarinetist, so her talent was not an issue. Opportunity, however, doesn't present itself every day. At that time, when the KU pep band traveled with the basketball team, just one clarinetist traveled.

During September 2013, I was covering a high school football game on a Friday night at St. Thomas Aquinas High School, just a mile or so from our house in Overland Park. I was on the sideline and

Aquinas was on an offensive drive. Right before they punched it into the end zone, Chase sent a text to Marlena and me. The band director at KU had posted a list on his door with the names of the musicians who made the basketball pep band. Chase took a picture and sent it to us. That's how she told us that she made the pep band.

As Aquinas scored the touchdown, I read the text, and I started jumping up and down on the sideline in celebration. I had a friend at the game in the stands who was watching me. Later he asked, "I saw you there on the sidelines. Why were you cheering for Aquinas?" I told him I was cheering because I just found out my kid had made the pep band at KU.

That started her real connection to and her own love of Kansas basketball. She's a kid who, as a junior in high school, couldn't tell you how many minutes there were in a half. Now, I can leave the room and come back during a commercial break. When I return, she'll say, "We're at the under-8 timeout and so-and-so just picked up a foul."

She's even a bracketologist. That's how special it has become to her. I love the way she has connected with Kansas basketball. She has found something, other than music, at the University of Kansas for which she has a passion. Even though she graduated, she stays connected.

On the day that she graduated, we were able to meet with the basketball coaching staff near the main drag on campus in Lawrence. They were taking pictures with the senior players, including Frank Mason. They allowed Chase and me to take pictures as well. That helped make her graduation day at the University of Kansas very special.

One of my two proudest memories was actually a time when I wasn't there. It was the day of "Late Night in the Phog" of her freshman year. Chase was in a freshman class at KU that included Andrew Wiggins, Joel Embiid, Wayne Seldon and Frank Mason. Thousands of fans were not allowed into Allen Fieldhouse for "Late Night" because there were simply too many people wanting to get in.

That afternoon I called Jim Marchiony, an assistant athletic director, and said, "Jim, I need a favor. Could you go near the pep band and take a picture of Chase before it gets too busy. There are going to be two clarinetists there. You'll be able to tell which one is my daughter. Could you take a picture of her and send it to me?"

He said, "That's easy. I thought you wanted me to sneak somebody in for you." When he sent me that picture and I saw her—and I knew she was not happy with me because she hated to be singled out among her friends—that made me as proud as anything.

It was almost as great as the day of the first home football game in September of 2013, when she came down the hill in that band uniform during the pregame. That was the best. With Chase being born in Lawrence and her affection for music, to see her march down that hill in that uniform was indescribable. It was an 85-degree Saturday, and those uniforms are hot and heavy,

I was proud seeing her as a Marching Jayhawk, because I knew she had worked so hard since junior high school to put herself in that position. It could have been any other school, and it would have been *almost* the same thing. She had chased that dream. She's always wanted to be a high school band director ever since the seventh grade. For her to take the next step toward that goal, at the same stadium where Marlena and I had met, that was the best.

There's no basketball game, no football game, no sporting event will match the enjoyment and pride that I had with those two experiences.

Remember, F.O.E. - Family Over Everything.

CHAPTER 10

3rd & Long

WE ALL MAKE mistakes. One mistake I made was back in the late 1980s. While working one day at WDAF, and I got a phone call from someone at KPRS radio. I can't remember exactly who it was. KPRS is the oldest Black-owned radio station in the country, owned by the Carter family in Kansas City. The person on the phone asked me if I wanted a part-time job delivering sports for the radio station. I said, "no."

I was mistaken to think I couldn't have two jobs at one time. I had always thought that my talents should be strictly confined to television, not radio, and anyone who was working in radio could not do a credible job in television. I never really gave it much thought after that. I forgot that while growing up, my father took as many jobs as he could to support our family.

There is nothing wrong with having two or three, or even four jobs, as long as you're not doing anything illegal or wrong. As long as my work at the TV station was not suffering, there was no reason I couldn't do that. I knew there were some other on-air employees at WDAF who had side-gigs working radio, but I had never considered it for myself.

When I moved to Kansas City in 1985, I never planned on staying and ending my career here. Texas was home, and my career goal was to eventually work and live in the Dallas/Ft. Worth area. I was presented that opportunity in July of 1989, but only stayed for a bit more than a year. Working at KXAS allowed me to realize that bigger wasn't always better, and that I shouldn't confuse someone else's desire to succeed with mine. I didn't fit in Dallas, and I was a big reason why.

I worked at KXAS for 13 months and put 39,000 miles on my car. I worked there during the first year of the Jerry Jones and Jimmy Johnson era with the Dallas Cowboys. I covered the first football game SMU played when it returned to competition after suffering the NCAA's "Death Penalty." I lived at work, and I hated it. When I was presented an opportunity to return to WDAF during the late summer of 1990, I jumped on it.

After I got back from my short stint in Dallas in August of 1990, I got another call from KPRS telling me that they needed someone to co-host a radio show with then second-year Chiefs linebacker Derrick Thomas. Thomas wanted to have a radio show and they needed a co-host, someone with broadcasting experience, along with knowledge of the Chiefs and the NFL.

The show would require me to open and close the show, negotiate getting in and out of commercial breaks, and act as a go-between with Derrick and any guests he might have on the program. That time my answer to KPRS was "yes."

At the time, KPRS was headquartered at Crown Center in Kansas City, so it was an easy commute from WDAF, which is located at 31st and Southwest Trafficway, It also wasn't much farther away from home, because at the time I was living in downtown Kansas City.

Derrick Thomas was the reigning AFC Defensive Rookie of the Year. I was working at WDAF the day he was drafted by the Chiefs. He was the fourth overall pick in the first round of the 1989 NFL Draft. At the time, the NFL Draft wasn't as popular as it is today. It wasn't expected that every potential top-10 pick would attend the draft in New York City.

After they selected Derrick, the Chiefs told local Kansas City media that he was spending draft day in Las Vegas. He was at Caesar's Palace when the Chiefs called him to tell him that he was their top pick. After hearing all of that, I got in touch with my old station in Las Vegas, which was also an NBC affiliate, and we got Derrick to agree to speak to us. He even agreed to speak with me in Kansas City via satellite that night live on our news.

So, on the day he was drafted, Derrick Thomas went to my old station in Las Vegas. They hooked him up via satellite and I interviewed him on our 10 o'clock sportscast that night.

That's how I met Derrick Thomas. He never saw me, and I saw him via satellite. I left for Dallas three months after that, and I didn't see him again until a year and a half later when I started hosting his radio show. A sign of things to come, sometime during that first month, Derrick was often five or 10 minutes late to his own radio show.

The radio show was called "3rd & Long," because that's when Derrick would thrive on the football field as a pass rusher. The other team's offense was under duress in a third-down, long-yardage situation. Derrick likened that to his connection to the community and the way he was brought up with a single mom.

His father was a fighter pilot whose plane had been shot down over Vietnam. Captain Robert James Thomas never returned home. Derrick would thrive in a third-and-long situation on the football field, and he wanted to help kids in life who might be in what's considered a long-shot situation to have success.

I've lived in Kansas City for 33 years, and I've never seen a player or a coach who connected with the community as much as Derrick Thomas did. He felt so comfortable in the community, just being with people. I felt he'd rather be there than any other place, being as comfortable there as he was on a football field. Derrick seemed comfortable in many settings, on the Plaza, in Westport, or wearing a tuxedo and accepting an award.

Derrick Thomas met the President of the United States, the late George H.W. Bush, and was named one of the "Thousand Points of Light." Yet, I believe Derrick was most comfortable in the community or in the library reading to kids on a Saturday afternoon when the Chiefs had a Sunday home game.

He developed his "3rd & Long Foundation" almost immediately upon his arrival in Kansas City, so it just made sense to call his radio show by the same name. To this day, the "3rd and Long Foundation" still exists, because it was something that he loved. It still has his handprint and footprint on it.

As dedicated as Derrick was to helping people, especially kids, he was the definition of a free spirit. He was a really good player when he was charged up; nobody could block him as a pass rusher. However, his hard work and dedication aren't the first thing that come to mind when I think about Derrick Thomas. Derrick was a man who liked to live day-to-day. His life didn't require much structure, and that's the way he liked it.

He knew he had to be at the Bluford Library Saturday afternoons at 2 o'clock, but he might get there a little late, because that's just who he was. Derrick was constantly late for just about everything. He liked to freelance, and as a pass rusher, that's part of what made him successful on the football field. Derrick wasn't the best tackler in the league, or even on the team. He was better as a freelancer. Chiefs head coach Marty Schottenheimer let him go on his own to sack the quarterback, and that's what he did best.

He was never, in my opinion, a great practice player Monday through Friday. Word has it, Eric Dickerson, a running back for the Los Angeles Rams was never good on the practice field. He saved his best for Sunday afternoons. Some players are like that. That was certainly true of Derrick Thomas.

Royals outfielder Alex Gordon is pretty much the opposite. He's the same every day. He practices hard. He has a regimen that he does whether it's the first day of Spring Training or in the dog days late in the season. He goes all out in his preparation, just like he does during the game.

That wasn't Derrick. He was two different people when it came to practice and the game. The similarity was that he was a freelancer on and off the field.

Here's a typical Derrick Thomas story. I got a call one day from BET, or Black Entertainment Television. They wanted an interview with Derrick. and they called me and said they would hire a photographer to work with me to do the interview with Derrick. The interview would detail Derrick as a football player, and his starting the "3rd and Long Foundation." They had it set up for a Saturday afternoon. We were to conduct the interview at Derrick's home in Independence, a suburb of Kansas City.

When we arrived at his house, Derrick was there and at least one teammate was there. Derrick had a crew that he ran around with, guys who didn't play football, guys who would run errands for him, or personally work for him. These were friends who did tasks like take care of his cars. He had one car with a license plate that said "Sack Man." He had another car with a license plate that said, "3rdLNG."

He had two or three cars. One guy on his crew would drive his car to training camp in River Falls, Wisconsin, for him. Then another guy would drive a second car. They would leave one car for Derrick in training camp, and both drive one car back to Kansas City. Later, they would go back to River Falls and get the car because Derrick was required to fly back to Kansas City with the team.

The day of the interview with BET, Derrick had some food catered in. He had a big sandwich platter from a local grocery store, which probably cost him about $100. It was a really nice spread, with sandwich meat, bread and all the extras.

We were all in the kitchen and Derrick had made an elaborate turkey sandwich that was probably about four or five inches thick. It had some mayonnaise and mustard on it, and as he took a bite out of his sandwich, a big chunk of mayonnaise plopped out of the back of it and fell on the kitchen floor, which had a real nice indoor/outdoor carpet.

We all just kind of looked on, not necessarily laughing, because of the big chunk of mayonnaise that fell to the carpet. Derrick just looked at it, then looked at us and said, "It doesn't matter, I'll just buy some new carpet."

That's kind of the way Derrick lived. "I don't have to clean that up, because I can just buy something new to replace it." He was not being arrogant; but to him it was no big deal, that's just the way he lived.

As a guy who grew up with so much structure, I wouldn't say it was hard dealing with Derrick's personality. It just wasn't mine. I noticed it, and in the long run simply thought it was harmless. Derrick was a lot of fun and he loved to have a good time. He was often called the "social director" of the Pro Bowl. Every other player at the Pro Bowl knew that when practice was over in Hawaii, Derrick was in charge of showing everybody a good time. He never got into any trouble, as far as I knew.

His best friend in some ways was Chiefs general manager, Carl Peterson. They admired each other a lot. They went to dinner once a week. They had always had that dinner date, though I can't remember if it was a specific day of the week,

Chiefs defensive end Neil Smith used to call Carl Peterson, "Derrick's Daddy." He'd say to Derrick, "There's your Daddy," or "I saw your Daddy on TV last night." Derrick and Neil were real close too.

When Derrick passed away, very few people took it as hard as Carl Peterson did.

In comparison to recent Kansas City sports heroes, say for instance Eric Hosmer or Patrick Mahomes, Derrick was totally different. For example, Eric Hosmer could go down to Kansas City's Power & Light District and buy everybody a drink after a big game. But when he walked out of that establishment, I don't know if anyone followed Eric.

Derrick was more of a Pied Piper. Derrick wanted to blend in off the field, all the time. After his radio show was over, he would sit with the crowd who had gathered and was just one of the people. He wanted to be one of the people in the community too. It's like he was saying, "I'm just like you because that's how I grew up. I grew up where you are." That never left him. That was always a part of him.

Nobody liked Derrick being late as often as he was, but it was part of who he was. In regard to his radio show, he wasn't late every week—but it was his radio show. Sometimes he would call in and say, "I'll be there in three minutes, I'm pulling into the parking lot." We'd go to commercial break and when we'd come back, he'd be sitting there. It never got to the point where we had to have an intervention with Derrick.

I pride myself on being a journalist, but the radio show offered very little journalism. All I did was take calls and intro and lead out of the show. That's one thing that made it a lot of fun. Derrick would never have a problem getting a teammate on the show as a guest, and he could always get a player from another NFL team to call in as a guest. They were glad to come on his show, because he would go on their show.

What's sad was that Derrick was part of the radio show for only four or five years before he went to another radio station. We then had to change the name of the show to "The Chiefs Hour."

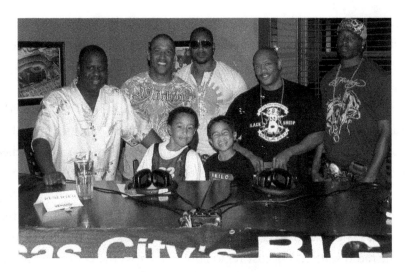

Al's involvement with the KPRS radio show lasted long after Derrick
Thomas left, including hosting with Eddie Kennison—second from left

There is an unwritten rule in broadcasting: you never ask how
much money a co-worker makes. I always thought it was none of my
business how much money they were making, and it's none of their
business how much I made. You don't talk about salaries around the
office, or at least, I never thought we should. I don't know if the other
radio station offered Derrick more money, but I did know it wasn't any
of my business.

After Derrick left, Neil Smith was the headliner on the show. After
Neil became a free agent and went to Denver, it was Donnell Bennett
and Danan Hughes. That duo worked well together. Then for a while
it was Eddie Kennison, and finally it was Derrick Johnson.

"The Chiefs Hour" went on for more than a decade. The program
ended when Carl Peterson's tenure as general manager with the team
ended after the 2008 season.

Two other interesting things about Derrick: first, he, just like me,
was fascinated by the assassination of John F. Kennedy. Secondly,
Derrick was born on January 1, 1967, on the same day the Chiefs won

the AFL championship game over the Buffalo Bills, to advance to the first Super Bowl. The Bills had a special-teams player by the name of Marty Schottenheimer, who turned out to be Derrick's head coach during his first 10 seasons with the Chiefs.

I'm thankful to Derrick for indirectly leading me into the relationship with KPRS. By the time Derrick left, I was established enough that they kept me on as the host. Eventually I was approached by the radio station to deliver sports during their morning drive time.

As much as anything, the radio station helped me enhance my connection to the Black community of Kansas City. It was my time with KPRS that allowed that relationship to blossom. The significance of the radio station, not just regionally but across the country—KPRS and Carter Broadcasting are well-known when it comes to Black broadcasters—opened that door for me.

I always felt I was hired at KPRS because I am Black. I was qualified for the job because of my years in television sports, but I was able to stay on because of my relationship with the people there. It helped fill my connectivity to the Black community in Kansas City.

The other thing that helped was the radio station felt I was very connected to the Chiefs. WDAF had built a strong relationship with the Kansas City Chiefs. For years, in the mid-90s and into the 2000s, we had the TV contract for the Chiefs preseason games. I wasn't Derrick Thomas, or Neil Smith, and I wasn't like Royals greats Frank White or Willie Wilson. I never put on a uniform in Kansas City. I came here as a broadcaster, not a ballplayer.

I had built up some equity and I think the radio audience realized that and appreciated it. In the mornings, when they introduced me, they would call me "Big. Al. Wallace." Former KU basketball great Wayne Simien once told me that when he was in high school, he'd drive to school and listen to KPRS. That's how he got his sports in the morning.

None of that would have happened without Derrick Thomas, and the need to find a co-host for his radio show.

I said earlier that nobody was as affected as much by Derrick's death as Carl Peterson. Just about anyone who followed the Chiefs was affected. Maybe part of the reason was the way he died.

The Chiefs had just lost to the Oakland Raiders in the Y2K game on the day after New Year's Day. Derrick wasn't thinking about retirement, but he definitely wanted to play in the year 2000 so he could say he played in three decades. To qualify for the playoffs, all the Chiefs needed to do was win that game against the Raiders, who came in with a 7-8 record and nothing to play for.

The game went to overtime, Joe Nedney kicked a 33-yard field goal to win the game for Oakland, and that eliminated the Chiefs from the playoff race. In that game, Derrick Thomas had recorded his first NFL interception. It would also be the last NFL game he would play.

Derrick took a week or so off, and then later in the month, was on his way to the airport to fly to St. Louis to see the Rams host the Tampa Bay Buccaneers in the NFC Championship Game. It was an icy and snowy day, and Derrick was running late, again. Gunther Cunningham, who had been promoted from defensive coordinator to head coach prior to that season, had told him for years, "Derrick, one day you're going to be late for your own funeral."

Derrick was driving his Suburban with a snake emblem on the side of it: we all called it the "Snakemobile"—and he was running late. The vehicle slid on a patch of ice and rolled over a couple of times. Derrick was thrown from the vehicle. There were four people in the vehicle, and only one person had his seatbelt on.

It was a Sunday afternoon and I was at work. I was sitting there with Frank Boal, when Frank got a phone call from a guy he knew at the NBC station in Buffalo. The guy from Buffalo said, "I just got a call from my nephew, who lives in Kansas City and works at a hospital in North Kansas City. He said they just brought in an injured person from an automobile accident, who he believes to be a player for Kansas City Chiefs."

He told us who it was, and we were in shock. We called the hospital and checked it all out. It was before halftime of the NFC Championship game, which WDAF was airing locally. We made a couple of phone calls and confirmed that it was Derrick Thomas. We had to do a half-time cut in, and report that Derrick Thomas had been injured in a single-car accident.

Someone at the hospital had told us it was serious, and it was confirmed the next morning that the injuries were very serious. Within 48 hours Derrick Thomas was flown from Kansas City to Miami. I was part of a four-person crew from our station who flew to Miami right after Derrick arrived. I flew with Meryl Lin McKean, our medical reporter, and two photographers.

There was a press conference there that day. Neil Smith was there. Derrick's mother was there. I knew both of them very well. Carl Peterson was there. I'm not sure but I think we were the only Kansas City TV station there.

It was heartbreaking, because they told us at the press conference how serious it was. He basically couldn't move from the neck down and the injuries appeared to be permanent. Marc Buoniconti was there. He is the son of NFL Hall of Famer Nick Buoniconti, and he had suffered an injury similar to Derrick's while playing college football. I remember interviewing Neil Smith and Marc Buoniconti.

We were there a day and a half, then flew back to Kansas City. Two weeks later, on February 8, 2000, Derrick passed away. He died from a blood clot that had developed in his paralyzed legs and traveled to his lungs, causing a pulmonary embolism.

We had to fly back down to south Florida for the funeral. There was a boat show in Miami, so all the hotel rooms and all the flights were booked. We had to fly to Tampa, rent a car and drive for four or five hours to get to Miami. We had to do the same thing coming back.

Marty Schottenheimer, who was no longer the Chiefs head coach, was there. Former Chiefs defensive coordinator Bill Cowher was there. Cowher was Derrick's position coach during those early years in

Kansas City. A couple of other notables were there, along with a lot of teammates. I remember Donnell Bennett, a Miami native, was part of the program at the service. He barely got through it.

There was a service for him here in Kansas City before the funeral in Miami, a service where I interviewed Hank Williams Jr. Celebrities came from all over to celebrate his life, because Derrick Thomas transcended sports. He had a lot of Hollywood friends, and Nashville friends because he liked country music.

I've never seen Kansas City mourn the loss of a sports star the way that Kansas City mourned the loss of Derrick Thomas. This city was down. The loss of Royals pitcher Yordano Ventura comes close, and we've lost others, but I don't remember mourning and hurting the way Kansas City hurt when Derrick Thomas passed away.

Personally, I lost a friend. I wasn't one of his entourage, but I definitely considered him a friend.

I cried. I called my brother Stephan when I found out Derrick had passed away. I was home and I had to rush to the TV station to be on the air for special coverage. I remember driving to work, and I was just bawling. I said to my brother, "Man, I love you. Don't ever take a day for granted. Not one single day. Nothing is promised. This guy had everything and he lost it all."

Mike Tillis was one of Derrick's closest friends, and he was a friend of mine too. He helped Derrick manage his day-to-day life as much as anybody. Mike Tillis died in that car wreck, just because he didn't have his seatbelt on. As I told my brother, nothing is promised, and we shouldn't take a single day for granted. You can be larger than life, and the very next minute, life itself can be gone. Derrick Thomas was just so much larger than life.

To this very day I still have a Derrick Thomas #58 button in my car right above my visor. The first thing I do when I get in my car is look at that button and remember "The Sack Man."

Then, I buckle my seatbelt.

CHAPTER 11

WDAF Sports

I SPENT A majority of my years in sports broadcasting at WDAF-TV in Kansas City—33 of my 40 years were spent sharing the stories of Kansas City sports on the oldest and most trusted television station in the Midwest. I covered the Royals, the Chiefs, Sporting KC, KU, K-State, Mizzou, NASCAR, minor league teams and a whole lot of high school sports, just to name a few.

I can't begin to count how many people impacted my life in my 33 years there, but I want to spend some time talking about my relationship with many of the people you probably came to know through the years, most of them on the air.

For the first 24 of those 33 years, I worked with and for Frank Boal. Frank was our sports director and our leader. To be a director or a leader in any industry, a person has to have confidence in their ability to lead. Frank certainly had that.

You could be in a room with Frank and any or all of the other people who worked in sports during my 33 years, including Gordon Docking, Denny Trease, Kevin Kietzman, Todd Leabo, Jason Lamb and me, and nine out of 10 people would immediately point at Frank and say, "That guy's the boss."

I'll spend a lot of time talking about Frank in the next chapter.

When I started at WDAF, the first person I met in the sports department was Gordon Docking. Gordon loved high school football and, other than the Royals and the Chiefs, I believe that's where his focus was. Having grown up in the Kansas City area and gone to high school here, Gordon had extensive knowledge of the history of sports in Kansas City. It's a factor in sports coverage that can never be overlooked. Knowledge of the landscape of any area of concern or coverage is invaluable.

Gordon had one of my all-time favorite lines while covering sports in Kansas City. The 1987 Major League Baseball season featured Bo Jackson playing for the Kansas City Royals and the Los Angeles Raiders of the NFL. Anyone who follows NFL rivalries knows the Raiders are the arch rivals of the Kansas City Chiefs.

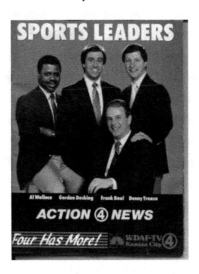

WDAF has a proud tradition of sports broadcasters

When the Raiders met the Chiefs at Arrowhead Stadium that season, Bo Jackson had arranged for a number of his Royals teammates to have sideline passes for the football game. In his opening line of his postgame report after the game, Gordon said, "It was the strangest thing I'd ever seen. The Chiefs were on one sideline, and the Royals were on the other!"

To think of a line like that took creativity and the ability to connect Kansas City's two favorite sports teams. He also never mentioned Bo Jackson. It was brilliant.

I admired Gordon a lot, because I think he was the first sports reporter in Kansas City to give the coverage of high school sports, especially high school football, the headline that it deserved. So much so, the Greater Kansas City Coaches Association created an award called the "Gordon Docking Award," which annually goes to a member of the media for outstanding high school coverage. In 2009, I was honored to receive the "Gordon Docking Award."

Perhaps the most valuable lesson I learned from Gordon, a lesson he might not even know he passed along to me, was the importance of community involvement. It's something I never considered in my first decade working in television. I was blind to it. Gordon didn't advertise the fact that he was continually involved with community work. He simply let his work speak for itself, and it spoke volumes.

The original cast of our sports department in 1985 also included Denny Trease. Before Denny was the play-by-play voice of the Royals, he was the play-by-play voice of the University of Kentucky.

They were both big jobs and Denny handled both of them with class and professionalism. Denny was talented. That was the first time I had ever worked closely with a play-by-play guy for a major sport or with a major team.

Everything was just so easy for Denny. I don't ever remember seeing him upset. He was always easy-going, even keel. You'd hear his call, and he'd be excited, but he was never over the top. He was just professional.

Due to the demands of a major league baseball schedule, Denny spent most of the year out of the office. WDAF carried the Royals games, and that was a seven-day-a-week gig from February through sometime in October. I truly enjoyed the time I did work with Denny.

The first summer intern I worked with in 1985 was Kevin Kietzman. Kevin was enrolled in school at K-State, and he started interning almost immediately after I came here. If he wasn't the very best intern, he was right up there in the top three, and that includes more than 20 years of interns. I'm talking dozens and dozens of interns.

Kevin knew sports and Kevin knew Kansas City. The only thing more dear to him than K-State athletics was Kansas City and the local sports community. He graduated from Shawnee Mission North, and he had the attitude of "Don't mess with Kansas City."

Kevin took me to the first BBQ place I ever visited in Kansas City. During that first summer in Kansas City, I didn't know my way around much, and Kevin took me to Haywards BBQ near College Boulevard and Antioch.

After he interned for WDAF, Kevin worked in Joplin for a couple of years. We later created a job for a sports producer that allowed him to move back here and take that job. He was the only one I would have recommended.

Kevin explained the lay of the land of Kansas City sports television to me. He explained that WDAF was considered the Royals station, and KCTV was considered the Chiefs station. At the time, the Chiefs games were seldom sold out, so their home games weren't on local TV. KCTV had the contract to air the preseason games. The Royals were usually the bigger sports story in town, and we had the Royals.

He explained as much to me about the local sports landscape as Frank did. I look back on it now, and I think it's because Kevin was wired in. The first day he worked, we assigned him to go to the ballpark. I said, "Make sure you get a soundbite from George Brett." He came back and had postgame with George Brett.

Another person who might be familiar to a lot of people in Kansas City is Todd Leabo. Leabo interned at WDAF while I was in Dallas, so

I never knew him as an intern. He joined our staff in the early 1990s, and I worked with him for about five years. Frank told me once that Leabo is the smartest man he's ever known. I didn't say the smartest sports guy or the best sports producer. Frank said, "the smartest man." Todd Leabo, in my opinion and Frank's too, could beat anybody at Trivial Pursuit.

He just knows everything. He knows facts, figures and dates. Most importantly, he knows the value of people, relationships and family. He's as knowledgeable a sports person as you will ever meet.

Most Royals fans will remember Paul Splittorff as the tall left-handed pitcher who still holds many Royals pitching records. But he was so much more than that. I didn't work with Splitt much when he was part of the staff at WDAF doing Royals games. He'd also come in and help with our high-school football coverage. That would kind of help him transition away from baseball on television and cover some other sports.

I was fortunate to work with Splitt away from WDAF, as part of the Big 12 college basketball broadcasts. On the wall in my office at home, I still have a framed press release, dated February 16, 1999. I did sidelines at a KU basketball game versus K-State at Allen Fieldhouse. The release said, "Fred White on play-by-play, Paul Splittorff on color commentary and Al Wallace on the sideline." That press release is a treasure to me.

Splitt was so much fun. He always knew that the game he was covering was just secondary to the game of life. He never took those games too seriously. I was always impressed by the fact that he knew college basketball so well, and he could connect with the audience at whatever level they were.

Whether they were a high-maintenance college fan or somebody who didn't know what was going on, he knew how to connect with them. Off-camera, he could tell stories about the old Royals and the current Royals. Paul Splittorff was just such a good person. It was a heartbreaker when he passed away after a battle with cancer.

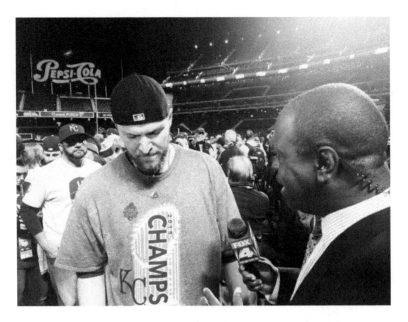

Al has covered a lot of successful sports teams, including the
2015 World Series champion Kansas City Royals

My last 16 years at WDAF, I worked with KU grad Jason Lamb. Jason came aboard in 2002. He filled a vacancy left by Ann Carroll, and just barely got aboard because news director Mike McDonald told us if we didn't hire someone that day, we weren't going to be able to hire anybody.

Jason was our first choice. He was a native of Great Bend, Kansas, but had been working in Topeka, so it was an easy hire. He was a Kansas guy, so he knew the local sporting landscape. He knew the ballparks, the Royals, the Chiefs, and he knew the coverage. He also knew the importance of high school coverage. He just fit.

No television news or sports department can succeed without good photographers, and one of the best was Don Proctor. Don is a lunch-pail guy. He went to Winnetonka High School, and he's a University of Missouri grad. I said this on my last day of working at WDAF. I worked with that guy for the better part of 33 years, and I asked him to do literally a million things. He never once said "No." Not once.

In the old days, Mike DeArmond was with *The Kansas City Star,* covering Mizzou as a beat writer. I've said for years, including numerous times at the Kansas City Tiger Club, "If you want to be informed on what's going on with Mizzou athletics, I'd first go to Mike DeArmond, and then I'd go to Donnie Proctor."

In recent years, because of staffing and technology, we just didn't cover as many Mizzou games. There are numerous factors that have contributed to WDAF not covering Mizzou the way we used to, or the way I thought we should. It's the biggest school in the state, a part of SEC football, and Donnie was our connection.

In 33 years at WDAF, I spent most of my time there working with the men and women I just mentioned. For more than three decades, we worked together, laughed together and made sure we did the best we could to inform the viewers of WDAF-TV about the latest in the local sporting community.

We did the best we could every day, and just like the teams and the players we covered, we tried to win every day. I'm sure there are other television sports departments that can say, "We did that, too." From 1985 to 2009, there's no way they had as much fun as we had. Not in a million years.

CHAPTER 12

Frank and the Old Man

I CAN SUM up in one word how working with and for Frank Boal made me better: Responsibility.

When you're a part of a team, part of a sports department or part of a newsroom, you are responsible to three different entities. You're responsible to the public, you're responsible to your coworkers, and, if you have one, you're responsible to provide for your family.

If you're a news reporter, you're responsible for asking the mayor that tough question, asking the senator why he or she voted a certain way, or asking business owners why they operate a certain way or charge a certain rate for services.

As a sports reporter, you're the one who goes into the locker room and asks the coach why his or her team lost or how they won. Not everyone who attends a game has the obligation to do that. A sports reporter is responsible to the fans who paid to see the contest, or the parents of the student-athletes. Why is the equipment the athletes are using sub-par? Why is the team continually doing what it's doing on the field that's allowing for success, or failure? There is a certain responsibility that you have as a reporter, an anchor or a journalist.

With Frank Boal, we were held responsible. It was something we rarely talked about openly, but it was always a major emphasis. We were responsible for covering sports and doing it a certain way. With Frank, we were responsible for being to work on time, and we were responsible to do the work required. All those things I had grown up understanding and practicing, the things that were part of who I was and the fabric of me, Frank Boal understood and required.

Frank and I had similar backgrounds, but there were still differences. I believe a lot of my ability to see eye-to-eye with him was because of similar backgrounds. His father was a disciplinarian like mine. We never talked much about each other's father. It was just an understood thing.

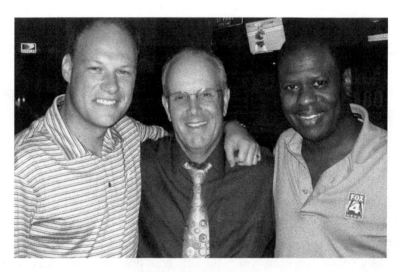

Jason Lamb (left) worked with Al for 16 years, Frank
Boal (center) worked with him for 24 years

I believe Frank understood the significance of Texas high school football. I knew the significance of western Pennsylvania high school football.

Frank played high school football in Pittsburgh at the same school as Dan Marino. Even earlier than that, he saw Joe Namath play high school football. All that carried weight with me. Frank knew that telling me those facts would give me an understanding of who and what he was.

Frank and Jan Boal were the parents of five children, so I could understand the importance of family to him. One thing I came to wonder was how he accepted being away from them so much. Frank anchored our 10 p.m. sportscast, five days a week for more than two decades.

From time to time, Frank would say to me when I was done with my responsibilities at work, "What are you doing here? Go home and be with your family." It didn't make any sense to him that two guys were there working late. Sometimes you have to stay late and work, and I never had a problem with that. When it wasn't necessary, he was always saying, "Go home, be with the family."

Frank, being the boss, had seniority in a number of ways, including having the first pick of vacation. His first pick was usually a week in July so he could take his family on a summer vacation. By the mid-90s, I got second pick. My first pick was usually the week that included Christmas. July was a bigger priority to him, so that allowed me to pick Christmas.

For years, my usual days off were Wednesdays and Thursdays. I always felt it was unfair for me to get Thanksgiving off, and to have the week of Christmas off. As the weekend sports anchor, I anchored Fridays and Saturdays. Frank anchored Sundays, which is always a big sports day. Since I got Christmas off, and every once in a while, New Year's Eve off, I didn't think it was fair at all that I'd also get Thanksgiving off, just because it was a Thursday.

Most of the time I would say, "I'm off Christmas, so I'll work Thanksgiving." I always had time to have Thanksgiving dinner early and then come to work late in the afternoon. Half the time we had a football game on the air, so we didn't have an early newscast. It made sense to me to be a team player; it was a no-brainer.

Frank not only taught the idea of sacrificing for the team, he lived it. We all sacrificed. It started with Frank. He would never ask you to do something that he didn't expect himself to do. or that he hadn't done in the past.

Up until the time he left WDAF, Frank did his own editing and writing. That was a requirement. We all had to know how to edit. We were all versatile. He required flexibility and versatility. That was the best way for our sports department to function. You had to be able to multitask before that term was ever invented. As I look back on it, I believe that was an excellent way to run a television sports department.

When he arrived in 1980, Frank developed a file system that still exists to this day. It has gone from video tapes to digital, but the transition was easy because of the way he designed the file system. The way he archived video tape, we simply archive digital media now. We could find an event easily because sports is all cyclical; seasons, and games, in each sport all happen every year, right around the same time.

There is a big difference in working *for* someone and working *with* someone. Frank's leadership style made it easy to do both. We all knew that he was the boss, but he didn't boss us. Your opinion always mattered to Frank. I could count on two hands the times he said, "I understand what you're saying, but we're going to do it my way this time." Even then, he did it with respect.

The first day I anchored a sportscast at WDAF, both he and Gordon Docking needed the night off. It was a Saturday night. Frank was going to some black-tie affair, but he dropped by the station real quick to make sure I was okay. He stopped by to read my copy and noticed my lead story was The Preakness Stakes.

He simply said, "I know where you're going, but this is a baseball town, lead with the Royals." He politely restacked my copy. I simply had to write it a little bit differently. Sure enough, five months later the 1985 Royals won the World Series.

A few months later. I anchored on a Sunday night and I included

NBA scores. When I started in May of 1985, the NBA Kansas City Kings had just cleaned out their lockers and left town, moving to Sacramento. When I applied for the job here, I wanted to work here because they had professional baseball, football and basketball.

The next time I saw him, Frank said, "NBA scores? We don't do NBA scores." He had the pulse of Kansas City. He told me once, and that was it. I didn't need to be told twice.

Most of the time, however, we agreed right away on how to do things, so he rarely had to overrule. And there were times, after disagreement, where he said, "You're right."

I remember when Bob Sundvold was fired as the head basketball coach at UMKC. Frank made a phone call to a source at UMKC, who told him that they fired Sundvold and they'd already decided to hire another guy. Frank typed it up for his next sportscast. I said, "What are you doing?" He said, "My source said this."

I said, "That's not enough. First of all, we need two sources. Do we actually *know* that, or do we trust this person enough to know that this is truly going to happen? This all happened in the last two hours. We haven't talked to any UMKC school or athletic officials. We haven't called this new person. Do we *know* that this is true?"

He looked at me and said, "You're right." As it turned out, UMKC did not hire the guy that Frank's source had suggested.

The point is, he trusted me. I'll bet when I first started working there, it took him 15 minutes to trust me. I can't sit here and tell you how much he was watching me, but he just trusted. When I first met him, he said, "You can edit, right?" I said, "Yes." He said, "Okay." Once he saw me edit a piece or two, he was good. That was it.

Frank had the ability, as a leader, to trust the people who worked for him, and that made it easier to work with him. To me, everybody in our sports department had a certain specialty. In a way, we were all just a different flavor of pie. Frank was the pecan pie. Technically speaking, maybe I was the chocolate pie. Gordon Docking was the lemon meringue pie.

We all brought something different to the table. It wasn't like we were all trying to get into the same space. There was plenty of room for two or three guys covering the Royals, but there wasn't enough room for four. So when Frank said, "Al, go cover some college basketball", I gladly took that role, because I didn't know what I didn't know.

I felt strongly that I was able to take orders. That's what I was told to do so that's what I did. Little did I know that it was those instructions that would launch my three-decade-plus love affair with college basketball.

Even though I liked anchoring, I didn't like anchoring as much as I liked reporting and producing. I never wanted to be the quarterback, or the head coach, in the sports department. I would much rather be an offensive or defensive coordinator than the head coach.

I loved working with Frank as support for him, more than I liked the last nine and a half years of working without Frank, where I was the main sports anchor.

I loved producing Chiefs Game Day with Frank and Mitch Holthus as the anchors, or with Frank and Kevin Harlan as the anchors. I loved working production and being a producer, building a 30-minute or hour-long show or setting up coverage for an All-Star Game. I loved cultivating the foundation of the show, because that's where my roots were.

Frank let me do all those things, and even relied on me to do those things. He enjoyed the fact that I took the responsibility of producing a sports program, which allowed him to perform other functions.

I don't know of many employees who could say they were actually proud of their boss, and the way that they performed at a certain point in time, but I had a tremendous sense of pride in Frank on several occasions.

One came in July of 1999, when Royals Hall of Famer George Brett was inducted into the Baseball Hall of Fame in Cooperstown, New York. Frank had worked for seven months to set up our coverage of that special day, because he made no secret that George Brett was his favorite Kansas City athlete. They were great friends.

On the night of the induction, after all the afternoon ceremonies were completed, the three other Kansas City television stations had coverage from downtown Cooperstown. Frank was doing live coverage for WDAF from George Brett's private celebration at a local country club.

During our late newscast, Frank had live interviews with George, his family members, former teammates and Royals team management. It was moments like that one that separated our sports coverage from the rest of the sports operations in Kansas City.

There aren't a lot of people in your life who get to see you progress from day one to the last day over 24 years. Frank saw all of that in me. He saw me as a new employee in 1985. He knew how I wept when he made the decision to leave WDAF in 2009.

I was sitting at home and I knew Frank had been offered a financial package to leave. He called me and I went out on the front porch, because I knew I would get emotional. I knew that would happen for two reasons. First, it hit home that he was leaving WDAF, and the 24 years were over.

Also, I knew that, in all likelihood, I would be moving into that slot. I would have to work late five nights a week and I would have to be away from my family. My younger daughter Chaney was 9, and my older daughter Chase was 13. I wasn't looking forward to that at all.

Frank saw me as a single guy, arrive in Kansas City then leave for Dallas in 1990. I left here to return to Texas. I came back here 13 months later because Kansas City had become home. The thing is, I wouldn't have been able to return here if Frank didn't give the move a thumbs up.

Our friendship developed at work and carried over into life away from work. I recall his joy when his kids were born, and remember the pride he showed when they graduated from high school. I know he missed so much of their lives as they were growing up. Very rarely did he say, "I need you to cover for me here so I can go do stuff with my kids." He did it a couple of times, but not enough. It was just mainly that he trusted me, and we became friends because of that.

No doubt the best part of working with Frank was the fact that it was fun. There were times when I would be at work with Frank and we would laugh so hard I'd have to leave the room. There was rarely a day, over 24 years, that we were in the office together and we didn't laugh. We always had a good time. It didn't matter if our sports staff was five people or three people—it fluctuated back and forth over the years—we always had a good time. It was always fun.

News reporters, producers or anchors all knew that when they came back into the sports department, they could escape the heaviness of the news. They called it "the toy department" because you could laugh. They'd all come back and have a good time. You could separate yourself from whatever was pulling you down in news.

I could tell you of news stories that I observed in the field because I was on my way to or from a sporting event and the photographer got called away to cover breaking news. Those instances could break your heart, because from time to time, that breaking news was tragic.

I was always thankful that I worked in sports and I didn't have to cover that kind of breaking news on a daily basis. It wasn't easy covering Derrick Thomas' or Lamar Hunt's funeral. Those things weren't a lot of fun at all, but they were the exception in our world of sports reporting.

I will always treasure my friendship with Frank Boal. He was a boss, a mentor, a colleague and mostly a friend. Along the way, he was as close a friend as I've ever had in television news, just like JW Edwards.

It was easy with JW, first of all, because he is Black. It was easy to relate to him almost immediately. When I first moved to Kansas City, I didn't know anyone. My friend, Alfred White, lived in Overland Park. He was a Texas Tech grad who had worked in the Texas Tech sports information office when I was at KAMC in Lubbock. In May of 1985, Alfred White worked for the NCAA, which was headquartered in Kansas City at the time.

JW Edwards was the first Black person I met at work. He said, "Hey, on Saturday mornings we all go up to the YMCA in midtown and play basketball." There were a couple of other guys from work that played basketball, so this was a way for me to build a social life, playing hoops on Saturday mornings.

We played in a recreational league, and JW was our player-coach. He always thought he was a good coach, but I tended to disagree. Through work, and basketball, our relationship grew.

Within the next two years, JW got married, and both Frank and I were part of the wedding party. I had known him for less than two years, and he trusted me enough to be a part of that special day in his life.

JW and I developed a comfort level and a friendship that was obvious. He helped steer me in a number of different directions that helped me get acclimated to Kansas City. He would say, "Go there and get your haircut," or "Open a bank account here." Hints to get adjusted in a new city are invaluable.

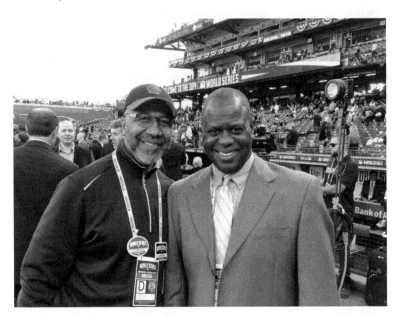

When you'd see Al at a sporting event, you'd usually see JW Edwards close by

Early on, I didn't work with JW any more than I did with any other photographer, so our friendship wasn't necessarily work-related. That changed when I made a suggestion to him. KU didn't make the Final Four in 1992, but it was obvious that it could become a regular occurrence. I said, "You're really missing out on Kansas basketball and the NCAA Tournament. You need to put in for that gig. I think you would really enjoy it."

In 1993 KU's NCAA Tournament run started in Chicago, then went to St Louis and finished at the Final Four in New Orleans. JW wound up getting video of KU "spitting in the river" in New Orleans before they lost to North Carolina in the national semifinals. That started JW's streak of covering KU in the NCAA Tournament, which ran through 2019. He and I traveled with Kansas in March during the tournament from 1993 through 2018.

During those 26 years, we covered 26 NCAA Tournaments and six Final Fours. We also traveled thousands of miles, by car and by plane. We visited the Civil Rights Museum in Birmingham, the Route 66 Memorial in Tulsa, the Alamo in San Antonio and the Muhammad Ali Center in Louisville. We also traveled to Bourbon Street in New Orleans and to the Lorraine Hotel in Memphis, where Dr. Martin Luther King was assassinated. Together, we saw all those places, all that history, while covering Kansas in the NCAA basketball tournament— all those places, and so many more.

Over time, we'd spend so much time together working, covering any sport, our friendship grew naturally. Personally, a couple of separate occasions stand out for me that personify or exemplify how much he means to me.

My daughter Chase was born in 1995 at Lawrence Memorial Hospital at 7 a.m. on a Sunday morning. JW is a church-going guy, but he was there right after the birth. I have a video that JW taped, showing me cutting the umbilical cord. He got out of bed on that Sunday morning in Overland Park and drove over, and he got me weighing my first-born. I have that precious memory because of the efforts of JW Edwards.

Then the next year, it was the October surprise snowstorm that came out of nowhere, where eight inches of snow buried the city. We were living in Prairie Village and the power went out in our house for three days. I guess we could have stayed in a hotel, but JW had a home in Overland Park with a big finished basement. He said, "Come on over." We lived in his basement for three days, my wife, our 1-year old daughter, and me.

Then again, four years later, when my daughter Chaney was born, JW again rushed to Lawrence to get video of me holding my newborn. It doesn't just work out that way by coincidence. You have to care. I can't tell you the countless times when I'd have concerns at work or at home, and I'd need somebody to lean on. The dude was always there.

We didn't agree on everything, and his expression was, "Let's not get sideways." It wasn't perfect, but easily it stood the test of time. When a friend can step up and take care of you in a family way, that transcends everything else.

A few of us at WDAF laughed at JW, because he could talk to anybody. There were times a coach would come out of his press conference for his one-on-one and you'd look around for JW. He was over talking to some security guard or arena staffer who, just like JW, was born and raised in Topeka.

I remember in 1997 when we were on the road with KU in the NCAA tournament in Birmingham, Alabama. News anchor John Holt was traveling with us. We were outside doing a live shot. John Holt had arranged for Kansas Governor Bill Graves to do a 5 o'clock interview with us. Governor Graves had made a special trip to Birmingham to watch Kansas basketball.

The governor walked up with his PR person, a security guard and a handler. He said to Holt, "Hi John, how're you doing?" Holt introduced me, and I shook the Governor's hand. Before I could say,

"This is our photographer, JW Edwards," the governor said, "Hey, JW, how're you doing?"

JW already knew the governor, and even more obvious was the fact that the governor already knew JW.

JW's presence and value transcended sports. He was, and continues to be, an ambassador and a representative of the station like no other. He started working at WDAF in 1978 and his career will go more than 40 years. My career was 33 years there, but I've got nothing on JW. It's not easy to do what he has done. I razz him sometimes by referring to him as "The Old Man." Sure, he's older than I am, but it's also a moniker I use with respect. Older most often means wiser.

Before I had the offer to leave WDAF, I knew he'd step away from work and retire in 2019. Part of my thinking in accepting the buyout and leaving the station in December 2018 was, "I'm not going to work here without JW."

I told former Kansas guard Greg Gurley at Kansas basketball media day in October 2018, "This is my last freshman class, and this is JW's last senior class." I knew JW was going to retire soon. I thought maybe I had three or four more years back in October.

A month later all of that changed, partly because I had no desire to work three or four more years in television news without my best friend.

CHAPTER 13

The Fight of My Life

MY FRIEND AND neighbor, Rob Mullin, was diagnosed with Grade 2 oligoastrocytoma—brain cancer—on January 16, 2003. Statistics at the time said Rob had anywhere from four to six years to live.

Rob, his wife Gail, their daughter, Holly, and their son, Gavin, had moved into our neighborhood a few years prior to that. Rob was employed at Sprint, whose worldwide campus is based in Overland Park, Kansas, near our homes.

My family had grown close to the Mullin family over time—my wife and kids more closely than I, because I spent so many evenings at work. We often would spend holiday time together, especially during the summers. Fireworks, Bar-B-Ques, it didn't matter. It was always a great time to relax and watch our kids grow up together.

When Rob was diagnosed with brain cancer, the way his family—silently at times—supported him was inspiring. We tried to be there for them as well. His biggest supporter was Gail.

Rob was a graduate of the University of Kansas, and he loved Kansas basketball. When he was diagnosed with brain cancer, Roy Williams was in his final season as the head coach at Kansas. Soon after, he left Lawrence and took the job at North Carolina, Gail made it her personal mission to make sure Rob was able to fulfill one of the three wishes that later would be on his bucket list: to meet Roy Williams. It wouldn't be easy, but Gail was determined.

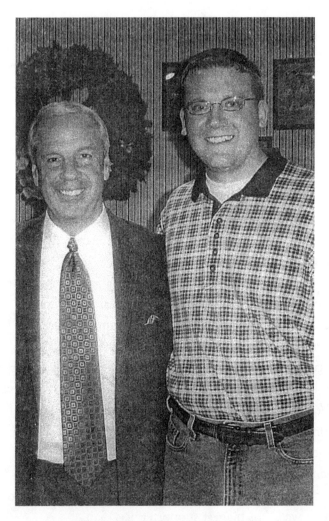

Meeting Roy Williams was at the top of Rob Mullin's bucket list

After some research and numerous phone calls, Gail finally made contact with Roy's secretary in Chapel Hill, North Carolina. Jennifer

Holbrook had a very sympathetic ear toward Gail, in part because her family had also been affected by cancer. Rob's treatment for his brain cancer would involve numerous trips to the Duke University Cancer Institute in Durham, North Carolina.

The campuses of Duke and North Carolina are less than 10 miles apart, so access to both campuses was no inconvenience when it came to geography. Gail hoped Jennifer could help in her request to have Rob meet Roy Williams during one of the times they were at Duke for Rob's cancer treatments.

Upon hearing that Rob was a Jayhawk, Roy rolled out the red carpet. He arranged for Rob and Gail to get a full tour of the basketball offices, and all the facilities connected to the Dean E. Smith Center in Chapel Hill.

Gail later would say that two details stood out to her during their visit with Roy Williams. First, the shower heads in the locker rooms where mounted so high on the walls. "Well of course they were," she thought. "They were mounted high for Tar Heel basketball players."

Secondly, she noticed the pleasure on Rob's face as he shared a couple of bottled Cokes with Coach Williams in his office. Roy had grown up in Asheville, North Carolina, and during his childhood years he had famously grown fond of drinking Coca-Cola.

A simple thing like drinking a Coke. That's how I remember Rob Mullin and his fight against a disease so dreadful and so deadly. He battled cancer for almost 14 years. I would lean on him, if only for a bit, in my battle against cancer.

Cancer has a significant history in my family. Both of my mother's parents died of cancer, and my mother eventually died of esophageal cancer, because she was a heavy smoker. I grew up with four sisters, and all four of my sisters had been diagnosed with some form of cancer. It's obvious that cancer was no stranger to my life and my family.

Right before my 54th birthday in October 2011, I realized it had been two or three years since I'd had a full physical. I went in for a full physical, and, of course, they drew blood. I left that examination a bit uneasy.

For my birthday, October 19, my wife and daughters treated me to a trip to Washington, D.C., because the Martin Luther King Jr. monuments had just been dedicated there. It was a three-day, two-night trip, and I went by myself. Marlena was working and my kids were in school. It was something I had engineered myself, and it was the one thing I wanted for my birthday.

Right after I arrived, I went to a Jimmy John's sandwich shop. I sat down with my sandwich and my phone rang. On the other end of the line was a lady from KU Med. She said, "We got your blood work back. We want you to come back in for some more testing." I knew then that I had cancer.

I went back a couple of weeks later and they did indeed find signs of prostate cancer. Doctors didn't know the extent of the cancer. They simply said, "This is what it is." I was at work when I got the phone call, and Marlena was the only person I told.

I've always told her and other family members, "If you've got bad news and it can wait until 11 o'clock, then just wait. If it's really urgent, let me know right away."

This was a case where Marlena knew I was waiting on the news, so I had to tell her on the phone that the news was not good, that I had cancer. I told her that doctors felt like they had found it early, but they weren't going to know for sure until they did a biopsy on my prostate.

The first person I told at WDAF was our general manager, Cheryl McDonald. That day was very vivid for me. I wanted to tell Cheryl first, because I was close to her and her husband Mike, and I wanted to start at the top. It was right after the Thanksgiving holidays, and I went in to tell her in a private conversation about 3:30 in the afternoon.

About a week later, I had a biopsy where doctors took samples of different areas of my prostate. The prostate is round, and you can have heavy cancer in one part and none in another. So they took samples from every part of my prostate, and the prognosis was that we had caught the cancer very early.

The plan going forward was to remove the prostate completely, having a surgery called a laparoscopic prostatectomy. My PSA level, or Prostate Specific Antigen level, was 4. My Gleason grade was 3+3 (score of 6/10), and I wasn't going to need chemo or radiation.

With timing and technology both on my side, I still couldn't have surgery until after my prostate healed from the biopsy. That meant that though I had the biopsy the first week of December, we didn't schedule surgery until February 2nd, two months later.

I've said numerous times that if God had said, "You have to have cancer. What kind of cancer do you want?" I would have picked some slight melanoma of the skin. Secondly, I would have picked the kind of cancer I had. The success rate of getting over and through it is very, very high.

After scheduling the surgery, the toughest thing to do was to tell my kids. I was going to have surgery on February 2, so Marlena and I decided there was no reason to tell them immediately after my diagnosis. If we told them right away, they'd have to wait two months and worry about it. Telling them immediately just wasn't necessary.

We decided to tell them sometime the last week of January, after we had gotten prepared. My surgery was scheduled for a Thursday morning, so the previous Saturday night we went to dinner. Chase was 16 and Chaney was 11. After we got home from dinner, we sat them down in the living room, and things grew silent. They knew something was up. They knew that a talk was coming. They had looks of, "What did we do?" or "What's going on here?" So we told them.

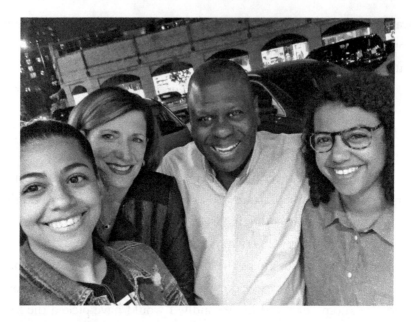

Marlena, Chase and Chaney provided all the motivation Al needed for recovery

They were both very familiar with Rob Mullin's fight against cancer, and what the entire Mullin family was going through right across the street. They knew Rob's diagnosis and prognosis, so when I told them I had cancer, they both just kind of sat there, stunned. We were able to tell them that my cancer was totally different from Rob's, and my prognosis was different.

Chase immediately just got up and went to the basement. To this day, neither one of the girls really likes going down to the finished basement by themselves. When they were little girls, they often thought, and we often joked, that there was a strange man living in my office down there. It kind of made my office off-limits. On that night, there was no fear of a stranger in my office for Chase. Her father had cancer.

Chaney went upstairs to her room, while Marlena and I just sat there. We turned on the TV and started to watch a college basketball game. Five minutes later, my phone rang. It was my neighbor from two doors down, Angela Kreps. I answered the phone and said hello.

Angela said, "Hi Al. How are you?" I said I was fine, and she said, "Are you sure you're doing fine?" Again, I answered yes, and said, "What's up?" Angela said, "I'm sitting here looking at Facebook. Chaney just posted something that said, "My Dad has cancer.""

I said, loud enough and slowly enough for Marlena to understand, "So you're on Facebook and you saw that Chaney posted that her Dad has cancer?" Marlena immediately ran upstairs. The first thing we said was, "You're 11; how do you have a Facebook page?" She said, "Chase said I could have it." That's how we came to understand that Chaney was social-media savvy. The difficult task of telling my kids that I had cancer turned into a bit of a funny episode. It helped break some ice.

I think it helps you get through difficult times if you have a sense of humor. If you are a worry wart, when you have difficult times, you'll worry about it. If you have a sense of humor, it's like, "All right cancer, bring it on."

My kids have always had a difficult time with illness. When my wife had a major surgery in 2010, both Chase and Chaney refused to go to the hospital. They didn't want to see her in the hospital.

After my surgery, they didn't want to visit me in the hospital, even though I was only in the hospital 36 hours or so. They didn't want any part of it. They even had a hard time coming into my bedroom seeing me laid up, knowing that I was basically immobile for a while.

I had the daVinci robot surgery on Thursday morning, February 2, 2012. I entered the hospital at 6 a.m., and the surgery started at 7 a.m. I was awake about six hours later.

When I was growing up, we'd go to the grocery store and see the vending machine with all the toys in it. You could operate a mechanical crane to pick the toy you wanted. The daVinci robot works in part the same way. The average prostate of an 18-year-old man is probably about the size of a super ball, or a cherry. As you grow older, your prostate grows. It's as natural as getting wrinkles or grey hair.

Back in the 1970s, 80s and 90s, prostate surgery meant cutting out your prostate by hand. With the DaVinci Robot, the doctor can be in the room or in another location operating the robot. Instead of making one big cut, they make five incisions around the abdomen, one for a camera. It's remarkable.

After surgery, I was up walking by 6 p.m., using a walker to walk down the hallway outside my hospital room. The next day, I left the hospital about 5 p.m. I walked to my car with help.

The doctor told me the first two weeks would be the toughest for recovery, and if I could get through the first two weeks, the rest would be downhill. I braced for the first two weeks to be a killer, and they were. Discomfort is the norm, and a normal eating schedule does not exist.

Most of the discomfort came from my abdomen, where it felt like I'd just done five thousand sit ups. I had painkillers and sleeping pills, but it was still a tremendous adjustment.

The two weeks went by fast enough. I couldn't drive while I was on any medication, which meant I couldn't drive, period. It wasn't good for me to even go up and down stairs. There were other adjustments I had to make in terms of bodily functions. It was tough and I chronicled all of that in a diary that I kept.

Monday, February 6

The kids are back to school today, the first day I don't have to take them. I miss it. Lots of "Giants Super Bowl" coverage. I don't care. I had a waffle and sausage for breakfast, lots of coffee. When you have the surgery that I had, the biggest obstacle is a bowel movement or to pass gas. The first sign that things went well and your recovery is beginning. And it may last a week, so there is a tremendous amount of discomfort...Oh, the little joys of life, a bowel movement. I got a call from Doug Tucker today. He recently retired from the Associated Press after decades of working in the region. We had a nice talk. I called him D-Tuck."

Tuesday, February 7

Doctors told me there would be days like this, down days. It's difficult to breathe at times. I get fatigued easily. There are still parts of my body that are taking their own sweet time getting better. That's the bad news of the day. The good news, Dr. Thrasher called this morning. Great news. Full biopsy on my prostate, only 10 percent of it was cancerous. Also showed that no cancer had progressed outside the prostate...I can now concentrate on my full recovery and not worry about my prostate, which is now history. I don't have pain anywhere. It is mostly discomfort. I try to keep it to a minimum, and some of the drugs and medication I'm taking help.

Wednesday, February 8

The key word of the day is routine. I seem to be settling into a routine. Is that good or bad? Too much TV and not enough reading of my Kennedy book. I am beginning to regain my appetite and continue to drink lots and lots and lots of water and it goes right through me. It means things are getting more normal, slowly but surely. I'm not claustrophobic yet. I try to stick my head out the door from time to time to get some fresh air. The weather outside is unseasonably mild.

Thursday, February 9

One week ago I had my prostate removed and now, one week later, I will never look at life and myself the same way. Life is too precious to be taken for granted. Even though we caught my cancer early, it was still cancer and no fun. Am I supposed to do something with this new outlook? Am I supposed to stand pat? Go it alone, with or without my family? These thoughts permeate my system. Am I nuts, or just human? I've known for months that I had cancer. At least for now, my body is cancer-free. What is my purpose? My brother, Stephan, picked up Chase and took her to school this morning. Chaney rode with the Kreps. Marlena has been fantastic.

Friday, February 10

This day was highlighted by two events: Susan Hiland called and we talked on the phone for 15 minutes. She's a great friend and makes a delicious salad. We always compared our salads at work. Fifteen minutes on the phone and I was never winded. She allowed me to do most of the talking and I explained my progress. She was a good listener. Chase has pep band at Olathe East today and when Marlena picked her up after the game, I rode along. It was my first trip out of the house in a week and it felt great. Fresh, clean, cold air—priceless. A trip outside the house that lasted 10 minutes, first time out of the house in a week. Is this a great country or what?

I always felt confident in the 90 percent survival rate with prostate cancer, but I had a resolve to do whatever I needed to do to make sure I was part of that 90 percent. It goes back to "One For The Coyotes." If the doctor said to do something, I did it, and then made sure I did a little extra.

My main motivation was my family—Marlena, Chase and Chaney. I wanted to be around as long as I could with them. I had a responsibility to them. What were they going to do if I wasn't there? If I had to beat cancer to take care of them, that's what I was going to do.

I approached my recovery from cancer with the same attitude I've approached so many other things in my life. I did it with determination and resolve. In other cases, I had a choice. In this case, with cancer, I had no choice. I couldn't quit. I had a responsibility. I hate to put it that way, because some people don't survive cancer.

Three of my best friends at work had survived cancer in the recent past, and I had no idea what they went through. I can't believe I didn't pay more attention to what they went through. I thought I paid a lot of attention to them. Sometimes I look back on it and recall saying to them, "Hey, do you need anything?" After my surgery I'd ask myself,

"How much did you really mean it?"

Before my surgery, I decided to keep a diary. I eventually talked about some pretty deep stuff. I grew up in a family where you simply did what you were told to do by people in authority. You could be human and question it in the back of your mind, but very rarely did you speak out against it. You basically did what you were supposed to do within the framework of what the Bible and the law of the land allowed you to do. That's the way that I was brought up.

When I was on a high school football team, my teammates depended on me to do my job. When I was working in television on a production crew to get a newscast on the air, everybody else was depending on me to do my job. You depended on everybody else to do their jobs too.

In the sports department, you have to do your job. That's the only way we're going to beat the other TV sports departments in town. On a team, you have to do your job; there's just no other choice. To beat cancer, I had no other choice. I had to do my job.

That winter of 2012 was very mild. We didn't have a lot of snow. I came home one night after I got off the air in late January. It was 45 or 50 degrees outside. I came home, and Rob Mullin was out walking his dogs. When I pulled in the driveway, I got out of the car and we started chatting. I told him how proud I was of him and how much I admired him and the way he fought.

I asked, "How do you do it? How do you do what you do? How do you beat cancer?" He said, "You fight it."

Rob was the mildest guy in the world. His wife Gail did all the talking. To this day, we joke about it. Those three words he said in my driveway have stuck with me ever since "You fight it."

He just made it sound like cancer was a demon. You get in the dirt with it. You wrestle it, you punch it, you kick it, you do whatever you can to it. You treat it. You may lose that fight, but you battle it. You help raise awareness, you helped others that you know have been affected by it. That's how you beat cancer. You fight it, and the fight never ends.

He was that plain with me. He was mad at the fact that he had cancer and that I had it too. He just said, "You fight it." That's all he had to say.

Rob's fight with cancer also made me realize that an attitude and awareness of extra effort, or "One for the Coyotes," could apply here too. It never hurts to tell those you love just how much you love them or care about them. One extra hug, one extra thought, one extra moment of caring goes a long way.

As much as I love history—and sports—I don't think either played a huge role in my recovery. I was fighting cancer, and that took precedence over everything else. Now, maybe some things I learned through history helped me stick to a strategy, like a general sticking to the plan to win a battle. Maybe I was inspired by stories of great teams overcoming obstacles.

I gradually regained my strength, as was expected. As the college basketball season went on, I had a target date to return to work. That was February 25, 2012. It was only a little more than three weeks after surgery, but things had gone so well that it became a possibility.

The reason that day stood out was that it would be the last time the Missouri Tigers would play a men's basketball game at Allen Fieldhouse. I knew I couldn't miss that if there was any way possible to be there.

The press credential requests for that game were monstrous. Talking with Chris Theisen, the sports information director at KU, I knew they were not going to have enough seats on press row for all the media who wanted to be there. Chris said a lot of the media were going to have to watch the game on a big-screen TV in Hadl Auditorium, in another part of Allen Fieldhouse.

That was fine with me. I've never been one to say, "Hey, I've got a bad seat." I figure I'm getting in for free, I've got a job to do, and there's going to be another game someday when I'll get a front-row seat. I didn't care. I didn't have to pay. I was fine.

As usual, JW Edwards and I got there early, because I wanted to soak it all in. I was back to work, and I was back at Allen Fieldhouse. As it turned out, about an hour before tip-off, Chris said, "I found a place to put you guys." I don't know where they got those seats, but I got a great seat for that game, three rows up from the floor, across the court from the Missouri bench.

I knew when I walked in that facility that history was going to be made. The air was thick, and you could feel the tension between the two teams. There was always animosity between the two schools, but on that day, there was even more than usual. It was obvious.

I could feel a rush as the Mizzou Tigers ran through the tunnel and out on the court. That feeling even heightened when the Kansas Jayhawks ran onto the court following a cheerleader who was toting a huge KU flag. You knew somebody was going to be able to brag about this one for a long, long time.

The outcome was going to hurt for the loser, and it was going to last. It was like that Armageddon football game at Arrowhead Stadium, when Missouri and Kansas were ranked No. 1 and No. 2 in the country, but for both schools at the time, basketball was more important.

Missouri led by 19 points with about 15 minutes left in the contest. Any flaw that that Kansas team had, Missouri was able to exploit it. Missouri controlled the game for the first 30 minutes-plus.

Of course, KU made the comeback. They got a stop here and a stop there and they cut the lead. That amazing crowd carried them. The key play of that game was a blocked shot at the end of regulation.

Kansas forward Thomas Robinson blocked a layup by Missouri guard Phil Pressey. It really was a foul; it wasn't just a blocked shot. Pressey should have been given free throws, but he wasn't.

The contest went into overtime and KU finally won the game. I remember Bill Self's reaction, right there in front of Missouri coach Frank Haith. He fist-pumped and his jacket almost came off. I've never heard the Fieldhouse as loud as it was that day. That place was alive. That was among the best college basketball games I've ever seen. I simply would not have missed that game for the world.

Since my diagnosis and treatment, cancer goes to the back of my mind at times, but it never stays there long. We lost Rob Mullin in late 2016. I was able to visit with him at a late point in his life, when he was no longer able to talk. He had told me a year before his death that he wanted me to speak at his service, whenever that was going to be.

We were at the American Royal BBQ once, and the Be HeadStrong Foundation For Brain Cancer Awareness had a tent. It was Rob's birthday, and I was honored to lead a large group of people in singing, "Happy Birthday." There were a couple hundred people there, and I did that gladly.

After being diagnosed with cancer in early 2003, meeting Roy Williams was the first item on Rob's bucket list. Meeting Bill Self was second, and meeting Bono (of U2) was third. He did get to meet Bill Self, during Self's second season at KU. Gail Mullin had contacted Joanie Stephens in the Kansas basketball office. Once again, her diligence paid off when Self agreed to allow Rob to visit a Kansas basketball practice. It was Gail's Valentine present to Rob.

Self allowed Rob, Gail and one of Rob's co-workers, Ravi Gargesh, to visit the team at Allen Fieldhouse. Halfway through practice, Self asked Rob to share his story of fighting brain cancer, and also asked Rob to share and explain his MRI. After the visit, junior forward Wayne Simien led the group in prayer.

Rob never met Bono, but Bono did write him a letter, three pages long. After Rob's death, in the summer of 2017, U2 performed at Arrowhead Stadium. Bono mentioned Rob Mullin in the middle of a song. He said, "Rob Mullin, if you can hear me..." One of Gail's friends was in the audience and just happened to be recording it on her phone, and it went viral on the Internet.

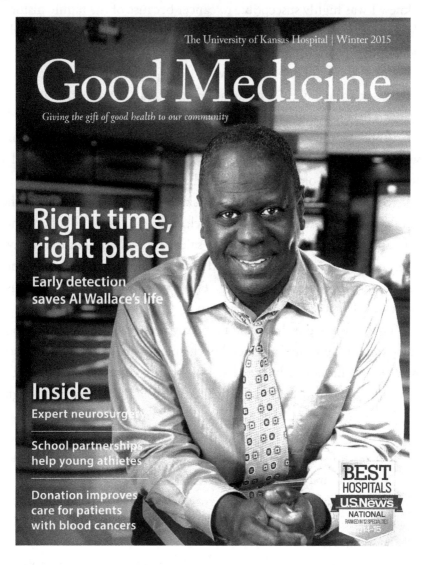

Al has been very willing to share his story, to inspire others to get early detection

Since my cancer, I've been fortunate enough that the people at The University of Kansas Medical Center have reached out to me. I've been able to tell my story in publications at KU Med, and a number of people have commented about it. I talk mostly about early detection. That's the easiest and safest way to get ahead of it like I did. I got a physical. I knew I was highly susceptible to cancer because of the family history. As a Black male over the age of 50, there was a likelihood that I might go through prostate cancer.

I used to get phone calls at work from people in the public. They would say things like, "I read the magazine article about you," or "I was at a function and somebody said, 'Al Wallace had prostate cancer.'"

People would call me and just say "What do I do?" I don't care what I was doing, I'd drop work to talk to them. I'd look up and I would have been on the phone with that person for 15 minutes.

In late 2018, I was at a KU basketball game, sitting up in the auxiliary media seats in the upper level, and a guy came by at halftime. He just started talking about it. He said, "I just found out that I have cancer." That makes me feel good that I can help, just talk to someone, just something that small: talking. That's how it has affected me; I just want to help others. Cancer is no fun.

That tough night that I had to tell my kids of my illness turned out to be something funny at the end of the night. I had no idea what they were going through. I knew what I was going through, and I knew it wasn't easy on them. I also knew what the Mullin family went through.

Before my cancer, over a 10- or 15-year time period, I missed two or three work days because of illness. After my cancer, I never missed another day of work at WDAF, because I always felt that if you're not sick, you shouldn't call in sick.

That final MU-KU game was the perfect way for me to end a one-month absence from work. If that's work—watching that game—I'll take work any day.

Here's how I wrapped it up in my diary, two days before tipoff:

Thursday, February 23

Maybe it's something you have a to go through to fully appreciate. The doctor calling and telling you he had bad news, and good news. The bad news is, you have cancer. The good news is, we caught it early, and the chances of survival are about 90 percent. After a lot of research and numerous consultations, we decided February 2nd was the date for surgery. "Don't worry," Dr. Thrasher said, "you'll be back in plenty of time for March Madness." I then thought, "There is a God."

The Madness this year starts a bit early, with the annual Border War game between Kansas and Missouri at Allen Fieldhouse in Lawrence, set for Saturday. This will be the final "on campus" regular season meeting between the two schools, with no other meeting scheduled any time soon.

Missouri is headed to the SEC, and Kansas wants no part of the relationship after the divorce. Kansas also wants to clinch at least a share of its 8th straight Big 12 Championship with a win. There's a lot on the line, and if you think I'm going to miss it, you're nuts. Not even cancer can keep me from being in the Fieldhouse. No way.

CHAPTER 14

Signing Off

NOTHING LASTS FOREVER. Not even a dream job. My decision to leave television at the end of 2018, actually dates back to the summer of 2009, when Frank Boal left WDAF. It's a dynamic that has hit television news, and a lot of other industries. It's that word we've heard so often over the last 15 or 20 years: "downsizing." In 2009 it hit home for me first-hand.

Frank Boal took a corporate buyout. When Frank left, our station management decided not to replace him with another employee. I will never forget the night in late June 2009 when he called me at home and said, "I'm going to take the buyout. I'm done at the end of the month."

I knew then we wouldn't replace his manpower, which meant a lot more work for everyone involved with sports at WDAF. Also, in all likelihood, I was going to be asked to move into his position. Instead of being home in the evening five nights a week, I would only be home two nights a week. That's what the job and the schedule would demand, and that's what eventually happened.

I was on the phone with Frank, and I didn't want my wife Marlena to hear the conversation, so I went outside on the front porch and sat on the steps. We talked for about 10 minutes. Afterwards, I wept. I didn't cry, I wept.

Things at work were never the same after Frank left. I always loved working in television. I always loved working in TV sports. I call it "40 years of my dream job," but the first 31 years were the best. It was still a great job, at a fantastic and historic television station, but it changed in a number of ways.

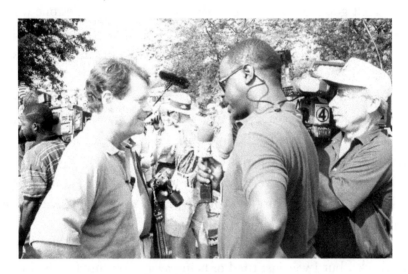

Covering all-time greats like golfer Tom Watson was
a regular part of Al's job with WDAF

Approximately 2.5 million people live in the Kansas City metro area. There are only about 15 or 20 people in this market who have the job of sports anchor or reporter in the 31st-ranked TV market in the United States. It was still a terrific job, but the absence of Frank Boal made it less enjoyable. Over the last nine years, because of the downsizing, it simply became *more* of a job. Still a fun one, but it just wasn't the same. The industry and technology have a lot to do with that, especially the way we would reach an audience or community.

Chase was 14 and Chaney was 9 when I moved into the lead on-air role in sports. I began to miss a lot of activities and time with my kids. Marlena had to do it alone, and that continually bothered me. The demands at work never lessened; they never grew smaller. If nothing else, because of the multiple ways we could reach our audience through technology, the demands grew greater.

It's nobody's fault. It was a simple product of the evolution of the industry. I knew September 8, 2018, was my 40-year anniversary. I always felt good about getting to that date. My next milestone would have been to work January 1, 2020, so I could say that I worked in six different decades. I figured working in five different decades in television news is pretty darn good--40 years and five different decades.

I've been asked a lot since my last day, December 20, 2018, if I wish I hadn't made the decision to leave. It's an easy answer: not one bit. I put it on a scale of one to 100 like this. I'm at 99 percent that it was a great decision. Only one percent was "What if?"

Recently while we were sitting down to eat dinner as a family, I said, "I just love this. I just love being with you guys." I missed so many things by not being with my family.

It's definitely a cliché: "nothing is promised." Every job has its drawbacks, but I was just tired of being away from my family. I don't know how people like Frank Boal, Phil Witt and Mike Thompson did it for so long. For years, they spent their evenings away from their families, away from their wives, away from their kids. I did it for nine and a half years, and that's a relatively short period of time, in TV years. When I worked in Lubbock, I was a single, young guy. That's called "paying your dues." That was a small sacrifice. This was a different sacrifice.

Some might think that one percent would kick in if one of the local teams wins a championship, but I don't think so. I decided in the late '90s, when Roy Williams coached basketball at Kansas and Marty Schottenheimer had some pretty good teams with the Chiefs, that I would develop no emotional attachment to any team that I covered because of work.

The Chiefs were 13-3 and were the No. 1 seed AFC playoffs in

1995 and 1997. I saw Dick Vermeil have some very good Chiefs teams too. I've seen Andy Reid have very good Chiefs teams. I decided more than 20 years ago that I should refrain as much as I could from any emotional attachment.

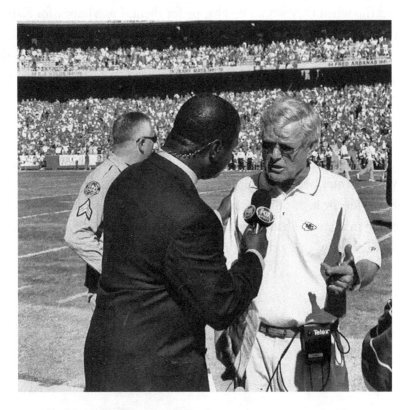

The Dick Vermeil-led Chiefs were exciting to watch. If only they could have played a little defense

I always wanted the Kansas City-area teams to succeed, but I never had a desire to cover a Super Bowl. If KU goes to a Final Four now, that's great. I'll be excited for them, but not *because* of them. When I was working in TV sports, teams winning or losing had both advantages and disadvantages. A local team winning meant more work, while a local team losing meant more time with my family.

I love the fact that the Royals, after 29 years, made it back to a World Series in 2014. They went to two consecutive World Series, winning it all in 2015. I love that. Yet and still, after 29 years of them not qualifying for one single playoff game, I refused to get emotionally attached. I didn't do a backflip when they won. I was happy for them. I was happy for Kansas City. I was happier for me when the coverage was over.

I'm still a big sports fan. I now enjoy watching games without the responsibility of having to report about them. I love it. It's the most fun I've had watching games in years, because I don't *have to*. I don't have to watch a game. I don't have to watch Missouri football or Kansas football or K-State basketball. I don't *have* to.

I still like to, but I don't have to. I spent 40 years of my life *having to* watch games because I felt the responsibility of having to know why a team won or lost, or why a coach made or didn't make a move or a decision in a game. I had to know so that I could explain it to a television audience. I now enjoy the fact that I don't have that responsibility.

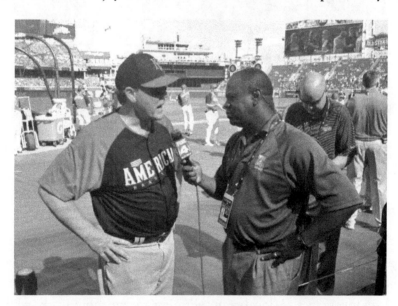

Ned Yost and the Royals took Kansas City on a
championship ride in 2014 and 2015

Let's say that KU and K-State both played a basketball game at the same time and Mizzou played two hours earlier or later. By the time I got to work the next day, I felt responsible for knowing what happened in all three games. Sometimes I'd have to go back and read about and research what happened. I had to be able to say with knowledge and understanding, "He dropped a pass," or "He twisted his ankle," or "He made that certain call."

If it's a game I do want to talk about, I don't have to limit it to 45 seconds. I can actually talk about it until the person I am talking to and I are tired of talking about it. An obvious difference is my audience is much smaller.

Early on, I described the role of television production as "game day" and "a rush of adrenalin." I've had plenty of adrenalin—40 years' worth. I got to work at the oldest, most trusted, and most respected television station in Kansas City.

I left Texas 34 years ago and Kansas City is now home. When I first moved here, I used to gripe and moan about how cold it was here, and how Texas was warmer and better.

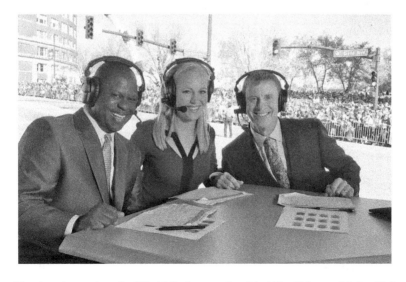

Al enjoyed covering the World Series parade with Abby Eden and John Holt

I worked here for about four years and then moved to Dallas. Then, a little more than a year later, I moved back to Kansas City. This is home.

I love history. I love Kansas City. My wife and kids don't want to live anywhere else. I got to work in TV—my dream job—in Kansas City for 33 years. I was the first full time Black sportscaster on TV in this market. Moving forward, and this is going to sound prideful, if anyone works in this market for 33 years doing sports on TV, I say good luck, and I salute.

Since my last day on the job, the question I get asked the most is "What's next?"

People in the grocery store or on social media, say, "You've retired." I haven't retired. I'm not done. I never thought I'd write a book, but now I've written a book, and I'm still not done.

One thing I love about history is the fact that history, itself, continues. Even after you're gone, your history continues in the lives of those you affect. After your passing, your history continues in your legacy, in what you did while you were here. Your history continues in the difference that you made while you were here.

Helping to raise awareness of early detection for cancer is very important to me. It's part self-fulfillment, but it's more a part of helping. To me, there's almost no greater joy than helping somebody who asks for and needs help. It's such an easy thing to do. I haven't quite wrapped my head around how I want to do that on a daily, weekly or monthly basis.

I am not sure of what is in store for me as far as a long-term future is concerned, but rest assured, I'll live up to my responsibility. People will depend on me, and I'll give it my best effort. In the meantime, all that work, all that attention, all that effort—"One For The Coyotes" effort—that I used to spend on television news, now goes into being with my family. It goes into loving my family and making them happy each and every day for the rest of my life.

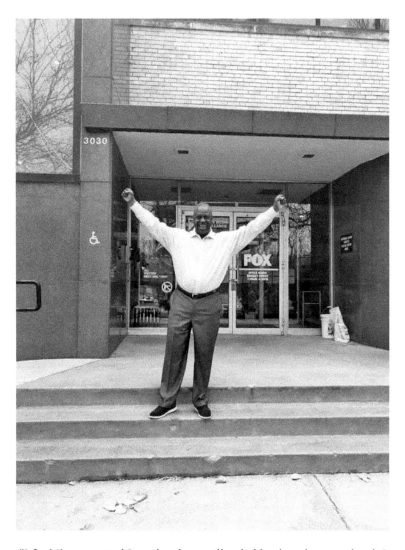

"I find I'm so excited I can barely sit still or hold a thought in my head. I think it's an excitement only a free man can feel. A free man at a start of a long journey whose conclusion is uncertain."—Red, from *Shawshank Redemption*